PRAISE FOR
Pain Studies

"Olstein offers readers an eclectic and deeply personal set of meditations on pain as experienced and remembered, inflicted and endured, perceived and denied. Through neuroscience, literature, and history, from hit TV shows to classical philosophy, this is a unique and fascinating contribution to the literature of pain in general, and migraine in particular." —**Katherine Foxhall**, author of *Migraine: A History*

"In *Pain Studies*, Olstein paints a sharp-witted and insightful picture of the rollercoaster ride that is called pain. Her own experiences allow her to approach the topic in a way that provides relevant reading to anyone treating or living with chronic pain. As doctors, we need to find more effective ways to help patients dealing with pain. This book is a step in that direction." —**Jill Heytens**, M.D., neurologist

"Like a prismatic series of artist's sketches, *Pain Studies* offers a dazzling variety of perspectives—personal, political, phenomenological, lyrical—on the unanswerable question of human suffering. Through virtuosic readings of everything from pre-Socratic philosophy to the trial transcripts of Joan of Arc to the cultural semiotics of *House M.D.*, Olstein brilliantly extends the literature of pain into our contemporary historical moment. But this searching work also illuminates how pain studies us. Turning the last page on Olstein's agonistic anatomy, we've come to know one of hurt's intimate acquaintances, unbroken by her suffering, or if broken in parts, then painstakingly remade."
—**Srikanth Reddy**, author of *Voyager* and *Changing Subjects: Digressions in Modern American Poetry*

Pain Studies

Lisa Olstein

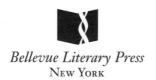

Bellevue Literary Press
NEW YORK

First published in the United States in 2020
by Bellevue Literary Press, New York

For information, contact:
Bellevue Literary Press
90 Broad Street
Suite 2100
New York, NY 10004
www.blpress.org

Library of Congress Cataloging-in-Publication Data
Names: Olstein, Lisa, 1972– author.
Title: Pain studies / Lisa Olstein.
Description: First edition. | Bellevue Literary Press : New York, 2020. |
    Includes bibliographical references.
Identifiers: LCCN 2018061040 (print) | LCCN 2019007332 (ebook) |
    ISBN 9781942658696 (ebook) | ISBN 9781942658689 (trade pbk. :
    alk. paper)
Subjects: LCSH: Pain—Patients—Biography. | Pain perception. |
    Pain—History. | Pain—Social aspects. | Pain—Psychological
    aspects. | Pain—Philosophy. | Pain in literature. | Pain in art.
Classification: LCC RB127 (ebook) | LCC RB127 .O42 2020 (print) |
    DDC 616/.0472—dc23
    LC record available at https://lccn.loc.gov/2018061040

Bellevue Literary Press would like to thank all its generous
donors—individuals and foundations—for their support.

 This publication is made possible by the New York
State Council on the Arts with the support of Governor
Andrew M. Cuomo and the New York State Legislature.

 This project is supported in part by an award
from the National Endowment for the Arts.

Book design and composition by Mulberry Tree Press, Inc.

Bellevue Literary Press is committed to ecological stewardship in our
book production practices, working to reduce our impact
on the natural environment.

♾ This book is printed on acid-free paper.

Manufactured in the United States of America.

First Edition

1 3 5 7 9 8 6 4 2
paperback ISBN: 978-1-942658-68-9
ebook ISBN: 978-1-942658-69-6

for David and Toby

and in memory of
Marion Daniels Covich (Annie)

Pain Studies

1

All pain is simple. And all pain is complex. You're in it and you want to get out. How can the ocean be not beautiful? The ocean is not beautiful today.

Pain is pain: vivid even in its opacity, vague even in its precision. Pain reduces and expands, diminishes and amplifies, bears down upon us, wells up within us, goes by *the* as often as by *my*, and only rarely by *our*.

"Fuck-fuck fuck-fuck" was when, circa hour seventeen, the doula knew I was fighting the pain rather than moving through, going deep, riding it, whatever—when she knew I would disappoint her. "I want to talk about an epidural now." My birth plan included something along the lines of please-don't-offer-me-pain-medication-I-know-my-options-and-will-avail-myself-of-them-if-I-choose. My mother always claimed she enjoyed giving birth and fought to do it naturally three times before it was the fashion. "How about we try the tub?" she asked. "Get me the anesthesiologist," I answered.

For nine months, I'd been migraine-free every day but two, a couple of hours, really, and mild, which was akin to a personal version of shattering the headache-free heavyweight world championship record. Colonized by plenty of other symptoms, my head—left frontal quadrant: check; right frontal quadrant: check; base of skull, top of scalp, lateral plane 1.5 inches down: check; eyes and eyebrows, temples: check—had been pain-free. Now labor pain was all pain, was all me. "Get me the anesthesiologist, please."

Later, I'd worry this is characterological, that I flee too quickly, too desperately into the arms of an immediate solution, be it Advil for cramps, migraine meds for migraine, epidural for this. I worry this tendency—weakness, fear, lack of imagination?—might infect my parenting, as well. I wonder if it's bred by the countless hours I've spent in uncontrollable or barely controlled pain, a specter always shifting. Not *if.* More like *how much* (a lot) and *how* (so many ways).

Perhaps you'll be relieved to learn, or maybe you've already guessed, that labor pain is not the pain I wish to discuss. The truth is, I couldn't. Seventeen hours and done—not the labor, but the pain, neatly ended by a spinal block—the blink of an eye, really; a memory, certainly, but one that draws dusky only a rickety bridge from here to there. Labor pain is like all pain, unknowable except while being lived. Fundamentally a creature of the present, physical pain remembered is by definition pain divorced. The difference between recalling the flu and having it—between expecting a child and having one—is like the difference between hearing a description of waves and drowning.

Drowning is one of the words we use to describe pain when we're desperately in it, though often it's used for other things, too: heartbreak, overwhelm. I've never experienced anything close to drowning, but I imagine that, like pain, it has a way of flooding you with the present. Yes, it makes you hazy, it fogs up memory's edges, but in the moment, it is the moment and you are nowhere else except and only exactly where it puts you.

In some ways like any acute pain and in some ways possibly unlike any other, migraine is a particular version of the present. What happens when its present becomes yours for extended periods of time, for a significant portion of your life? This is the pain, or the present, I wish to discuss.

2

———

Does the dark, early-morning skull shatter by the light of waking, or does the shattering wake the skull to dark, early morning? Either way, it's like an iceberg cracking, but within the cramped confines of a dumpy container ship. Today? No, not today. Rather, yes, today, again. "Small streams may become raging currents without warning," the National Weather Service's alert flashes on repeat. No shit. In other words, despite all the information at your disposal, you're not going to see this coming. (I never do.)

Whatever pain you're in is the worst kind, and when it's bad, it's untranslatable, but that doesn't keep you from having to try.

Masturbate forever, chanting "I am alone"
in Middle Persian

Dig through a hill with your breasts,
  wearing a millstone for a cap

Be thou a deathless thorn-tree in the suicidal
  woods

These are some of the forms of suffering listed on an altered version of the Wong-Baker Faces Pain Rating Scale to be ranked by the patient (that is, reader; that is, you) in a poem about the underworld by Srikanth Reddy. Hearing him read it—a finished section of an incomplete epic—shortly before leaving town for a residency that will give me uninterrupted time to write, I'm struck by how, ingenious as varieties of pain, they're equally apt as descriptions of what it's like to try to describe pain at all.

Pain as black box, lockbox, substitute safe hoarding vital data. Pain as memory's shrapnel. Pain as vehicle. Pain as avenue (spiritual, sexual, other). Pain as evidence of God's love. Pain as evidence of God's wrath. Pain as healthy. Pain as diseased. Pain as hollow attachment. Pain as deepest bond. Pain as symptom. Pain as cause. Pain as passing. Pain as lasting. Pain as telling, as smoke screen, as distraction's pesky fly. Pain as phantom. Pain as proof.

Dull, sharp, throbbing, burning, aching, stabbing, concentrated, diffuse. Infrequent, occasional, intermittent, frequent, constant, mild, moderate, severe, tie me a noose. Despite or perhaps because of the dizzyingly various ways we categorize and conceptualize (let alone experience) pain, we're notoriously bad at talking about it, even literally, as in, do you have it, how much, where, what kind?

"The sensations of my own body may be the only subject on which I am qualified to claim expertise. Sad and terrible, then, how little I know," writes Eula Biss in the "The Pain Scale." Before coming across the essay, I'd spent years hating the standard numerical scale—rank your pain from 1–10, 1 being no pain and 10 being the worst pain you can imagine—and hating myself when confronted by it, ricocheting as I did between indignation, shame, and confusion. So finding the essay was a kind of reprieve, the validation of a frustration that had long confounded me.

Looking for better systems of measurement, Biss points us toward the Beaufort Wind Scale. Developed in 1805 by Sir Francis Beaufort of the British Royal Navy (undoubtedly along with many unnamed others) to categorize the speed of wind, it runs from 0–12, but the numbers are the least important part. They read as shorthand, really, for exquisitely tuned, twinned descriptions of the physical world by land and by sea. Biss quotes several of the on-land descriptions—"wind felt on face; leaves rustle"—but I find it's what happens at sea that reads eerily like a mounting migraine:

Sea surface smooth and mirror-like

Scaly ripples, no foam crests

Small wavelets, crests glassy, no breaking

Large wavelets, crests begin to break, scattered whitecaps

Small waves becoming longer, numerous whitecaps

Moderate waves taking longer form, many whitecaps, some spray

*Larger waves, whitecaps common, more
    spray*

Sea heaps up, white foam streaks off breakers

*Moderately high waves of greater length,
    edges of crests begin to break into
    spindrift, foam blown in streaks*

*High waves, sea begins to roll, dense streaks
    of foam, spray may reduce visibility*

*Very high waves with overhanging crests,
    sea white with densely blown foam, heavy
    rolling, lowered visibility*

*Exceptionally high waves, foam patches cover
    sea, visibility more reduced*

*Air filled with foam, sea completely white
    with driving spray, visibility greatly
    reduced*

3

Embarkation, a present now months in the
past: I fly several hours across the vast state, am
driven several more under vast skies from a big
border city to a tiny border town, straight to
dinner around a brightly lit table. "What will
you be working on while you're here?" is where
the conversation inevitably turns. "Something
about pain," I say to these welcoming strang-
ers—a few people from the foundation, the
two other writers in residence—almost without meaning to. Given more thought, or given
less travel, I would have been more circum-
spect. Why? In order to guard the space around
the imagination, the unanswered, as yet even
unuttered, invitation for language to rise up, to
touch down. And because I don't lead with this,
ever. Despite all the evidence, all the years, I

don't identify—certainly not at the outset—as a person in pain.

Today? No, not today. This morning is another morning of waking into pain: left brow like a pressed bruise, an overripe peach you accidentally stuck your fingers into; top of head a china vase in a vise tightening, all angled echo and clamor. Sometimes a chisel striking, somewhere metal on metal.

Take at earliest onset of symptoms. Dependency may occur with overuse. Hold perfectly still sitting upright in bed whispering *no, no, no*. Wait to stretch, to drink, to log last night's meal into your possible food-trigger diary before reaching for the pills. Reach for the pills hours ago still half in sick sleep. Decide Sheetrock or precision pickax.

One doctor says I'll give you all the X you need. One doctor says your pain will have to be managed elsewhere. One doctor says you have to be careful, X is a dirty drug; they've outlawed it in the Netherlands. One doctor says X is one of our oldest and safest treatments. One doctor says X is okay, but you can habituate—does it still work?

Today? In Heather Abel's "How to Prevent a Tsunami in Three Easy Steps," this is the question framing a Santa Monica childhood preoccupied with fear of the Big One, the massive earthquake plus tidal wave widely thought to be imminent. "I'd stand in the doorway of my mom's bedroom and ask if there'd be a tsunami that day. She would say no, not today. This was our script." Narrow the aperture; return time to fathomable portions.

In my version, I've inverted the equation because I'm hoping not for the status quo, but for the miraculous anomaly. The question housed in my *Today?* is *Will today be different? Will today be pain-free?* The reassurance buried deep inside the answer *No, not today* is the best I can do. Fathomable portions. *Maybe tomorrow?*

Years ago, before the migraines turned chronic, a classmate's brother fell off a third-story balcony (darkness, drinking, no railing) and broke nearly everything. A few weeks later, my classmate turned in a poem set at his brother's hospital bedside that ended with a declaration of love's duration: he broke down into hours and minutes the length of time from his brother's birth to the poem's present moment of sitting beside him. Something in the calculation, its meticulous accounting in the face of faceless time, its insistence on the fact and finiteness of individual existence, has stayed with me ever since, equal parts beauty and dread.

My clock started ticking one fall morning in 1997 when I woke up with a headache that lasted three months, ushering in the era I inhabit still: acute-chronic, chronic-acute. Previously, I'd had one or two migraines as a child, along with a handful of auras—a sudden barred strangeness to the light, an accordioning of sound, an inexplicable drag on the time signature of a moment or an afternoon—understood only in retrospect. Between the ages of eighteen and twenty-five, I had what I've come to call "normal-person" migraine: occasional, stress-related, just like my mother's. Then, boom: days, weeks, sometimes months at a time.

Always the answer is "Many" to the question "How many?" over the course of any given swath of time. A cautious estimate for my current common era:

approximately 3,472 days of migraine, which is 83,328 hours (including sleep migraine-lit), which is 4,999,680 minutes, or, alternately, 9.5 years. But who's counting?

4

___

Red means cheap in contemporary advertising vernacular. When words for color enter a language, linguists tell us, they arrive first as black—which we're grade-school taught is not a color, but an absence—and white. Then red. For blood? Something visceral, having to do with viscera? Blue, they say, is one of the last to arrive, but this seems not quite right. Maybe we don't need to name what is so omnipresent around us (sea, sky)? Maybe calmness soothes us away from our urge to name it? Considered a color of mental clarity and deep spirituality, both, I've never heard of blue agitating or disturbing the mind.

Hovering between activity and passivity, excitation and rest, blue has, Goethe writes, "a peculiar and almost indescribable effect on the eye . . .

a stimulating negation." Maybe because of the expanses across which we perceive it (sea, sky), it can't help but be infused by that which falls away or is always far off. "As the upper sky and distant mountains appear blue, so a blue surface seems to retire from us." And maybe we can't help but find this elusiveness alluring. "But as we readily follow an agreeable object that flies from us, so we love to contemplate blue, not because it advances to us but because it draws us after it."

Kandinsky had a system, too, a synesthetic mash-up of personification, emotion, and sound. According to him, orange is a middle-range church bell, an alto voice. Green (middle position violin) is like a very fat, very healthy cow. Gray is soundless. Blue, when it sinks toward black, has an overtone of mourning that is not human. As it ranges in hue, so it ranges in sound, from flute (light blue) to cello (darker blue) to organ (darkest blue of all).

Personally, I want to eat it, but can control the urge. I don't think I felt this way about blue before migraine turned all colors all-body: the eyes absorb them as if drinking through a double straw, the nerves register vibrate or lull, vessels smooth or bristle, a concert of sensation loops from eye to stomach to back of skull, something deep in the arms starts to whir. On days when the lids are curtains often emergency-drawn, yellow is horrible. Certain greens pure sick. Red, no thank you. White, the nurse you don't want to see coming. Blue, though, speaks a language of no harm.

5

Before leaving for the residency that will allow me to devote several weeks to writing about pain, I leave a note on my son's pillow, shamelessly aiming for some expression of love that will tickle his seven-year-old sensibility but still hold true as an articulation of my devotion (in the meantime? for all time should my plane go down?). *I love you × 1,000,000. I love you all the time. I love you to infinity. I love you deeper than the Mariana Trench. I love all of you.* Every word is true, of course. How, then, to reconcile the feeling that if I had it to do over again, I wouldn't have had a child?

What I mean is, the pain of labor does usher in a longer-lasting and novel pain condition, that of loving someone more and differently than ever before and having brought that person into the mortal world—not just a world in which we experience pain and death, but a world that is, by our own most vital measures, dying. Every fear is recast: now the nightmare scenario isn't falling unconscious to the floor, not to be found, but falling unconscious to the floor, immediately to be found by your helpless beloved; isn't to suffer the nighttime assault or the cataclysmic storm or the devastating drought, but to suffer your child suffering—or witnessing you suffer—it.

This isn't anything new, but we live in a world with radically new and catastrophic predictions turned calculations quickly turning foregone conclusions, and having a child extends and condenses the math—your math. But a mother's love and fear in the face of ordinary mortality and looming climate catastrophe is not the kind of pain I mean to address here. Here, I have to remind myself, I mean to focus specifically on the physical kind, a subset even of that. (Each bird is one bird worrying one weak-shelled clutch of eggs or searching for the answer of a morsel or a mate.)

Strategic denial, cool compartmentalization, comparative abyss: I know the facts but can't stick my nose in them and expect to easily pull it back out. Every new work-up, every new full-history intake, every new megastudy or super-storm—rehearsing the years, aggregating the data—sends me circling down, so, increasingly, I avoid them.

The thing is, hope doesn't run the numbers on what falls within reach versus what remains beyond our grasp, so each time we start, we start at zero, and this is the rub. Over and over we may hope, but in doing so, sometimes we rub raw. For years, my biggest fear was that I would somehow unwittingly turn away from the one thing that would finally help me. So I kept on with my quest, kept troubling each decision with this fear not only of missing out but of somehow foolishly being the one to make myself miss out on my one chance at a cure. After too many hours, medicines, modalities, and dollars to tally, I still harbor this fear, but a new one has taken up residence beside it—not a fear, exactly, a feeling: maybe to keep hoping, to keep quest-ing, is its own kind of pain; maybe I need to stop.

6

The feline mouth is dirtier than the canine, so if you need a wound licked, better to go with a dog. Urine takes the sting out of jellyfish poison but not out of snake venom. There is a parasite that will cause a mouse to undertake risky, cat-attracting, even cat-seeking, behaviors. Intermediate host, the mouse dies, predictably and by design. The parasite moves on to its destination, the cat, in whose intestines the parasite's own reproduction occurs. What is the analogy here? A set of questions, I suppose: How do we feel what we feel and why? Play in the open, the parasite says, and the mouse complies.

After moving us into our new home, Kyle, a former marine turned long-haul trucker, planned to visit his eighty-four-year-old father for a few days in West Texas. "Dad's doing fine, still rides a horse every day," he tells us, "but he's not as agile as before the fall." He relates the story: His father, eighty-two, moving cattle one cold morning hundreds of acres deep. After trailering his horse up, he left the truck and rode. Near a gate, the horse slipped on some ice and fell. His father's back and arm were broken; the horse spooked and took off running. The old man dragged himself two miles back to where the truck was parked, the horse now grazing beside it, having run for the closest available thing to home. Somehow, he loaded the horse into the trailer and drove the two hours into town, heading straight to the livestock auction where he sold the horse before checking himself into the hospital.

Over how much and what do we exert control? *Influence* is probably a better word, control being out of the hands of the gods even, if you read the primary texts.

Lucretius, the first-century B.C. Roman poet-philosopher, about whom very little is known, came up with the term *clinamen* to describe his concept of creation: the unpredictable swerve of atoms "occurring at no fixed place or time" that makes all life possible. According to him, atoms typically fall in a straight and regular rain. Nothing happens. When an atom breaks rank with its sterile trajectory and collides with another atom, creation occurs.

> *But if they were not in the habit of swerving, they would all fall straight down through the depths of the void, like drops of rain, and no collision would occur, nor would any blow be produced among the atoms. In that case, nature would never have produced anything.*

In less luminous modern usage, the *Oxford English Dictionary* defines *clinamen* as an "inclination" or "bias." *Merriam-Webster's* offers: "turn, bias, twist; from the Latin *clinare*, to bend," before noting, "This word doesn't usually appear in our free dictionary, but the definition from our premium Unabridged Dictionary is offered here on a limited basis." In contemporary literary circles, *clinamen* is sometimes used to describe a writer's swerve away from inheritance or influence, or the act of deliberately breaking a stylistic or formal rule to enhance through disruption the beauty of a whole.

Chaos as design. Causality versus coincidence. Serendipity. Accident. Context. Prediction bias, selection bias, sampling bias, response bias, reliability, the law of diminishing returns. All pain is simple. And all pain is complex. 8, 24, 66: according to the index, the pages on which *migraine* appears in *The Story of Pain*. A bit thin, don't you think? 34, 35, 66–67,147,159–60, 162, 248–50, 283, 333, 359, according to the index of *The Pain Chronicles*. Now we're talking. In this index, Woolf appears and Hippocrates, Napoléon and Nabokov. Opium poppy, ordeals, orthopedists, Ovid.

7

"Have you talked about it with MaryJo?" Timothy asks when I tell him I'm thinking about trying to write about migraine. "Hers went away." Yes, we talked about it, so how can it be that all I remember is that she'd had them enough like me that in our eyes we understood we understood? Hers had gone away? Something vague flutters by. "It may have been hormonal," Timothy says. "Yes," I answer, "I think she timed out." How is it possible I could not remember this successful grasping of the brass ring, a parallel quest completed? I think we got sidetracked when one of us mentioned Joan of Arc.

Why Joan? The patient-cum-defendant endlessly examined, poked at and prodded, revered and reviled, the center around which the whole unwelcome circus spins. The subject forced to speak in and of the untranslatable condition of herself. The subject sure and unsure. The choosing between evils. I don't care about the church or Joan's relationship to God or the Hundred Years' War. I care about what she says. The expression of one's inexpressible experience for an avid but not necessarily sympathetic audience of nonpeers: A bit too often like doctor/patient, no? A lot like pain.

Why Joan? Because required to voice the private publicly, she often refused. Because she uttered the unutterable while somehow staying true to it. That is to say, because of her relationship to language.

Because she was a woman surrounded by prying, know-it-all, highly trained, deeply biased men who pelted her with questions, forcing her to defend herself for what was no offense but which offended them—their sensibilities, their sense of power and decorum, of how things went.

Because she heard voices and saw light.

Because, bodily, she did not behave. Because by insisting on what her body felt or needed, she defended it from certain kinds of attack while opening it to others.

Because everywhere I turn, my life is crowded with too many questions and too many answers, often in mismatched pairs, and frequently this is how Joan's testimony reads.

Because although she is so well known, so widely claimed, really, we know so little about her.

Because I wanted to start with nothing, or, in the sink and surge of migraine-mind, I found myself drawn to this crowded near nothingness: the intriguing cloud of potential and projection, the thrill of an almost unpredetermined chase combined with the shifty allure of a cliché's intentionally low stakes.

Or because I wanted to start with something I knew nothing about, but could have, should have, maybe once did. What do we learn? What do we recall? What does it mean? I was born to college-educated parents in the Greater Boston area in 1972. I attended "good" schools. The first time I learned anything about the Ottoman Empire was in 2003 and it was only because I happened to be studying in Greece.

I never learned anything at all about Joan of
Arc, except ambiently, the three-syllable beat
of her name.

8

———

Why Joan? Because recently, I'd been encountering mention of her in intriguing ways:

In an essay by Anne Carson on translation—largely, the impossibility at its heart—pointing to Joan's refusal to translate her experience into acceptable terms: "Joan wanted to convey the jar on the nerves without translating it into theological cliché. It is her rage against cliché that draws me to her. A genius is in her rage. We all feel this rage at some level, at some time. . . . We resort to cliche because it's easier than trying to make up something new. Implicit in it is the question, Don't we already know what we think about this?"

In an essay by Elizabeth Willis on the potential of language to both impose and resist aspects of oppression and domination, pointing to Joan as an example of each: "Saint Joan was referred to as The Maid. Even after she led an army. . . . Like The Maid, we have the right to transform the disciplinary structures of our world with sulphurous language. To fight one fire with another."

And in a profile of former UN ambassador Samantha Power, which early on describes her in reference to Joan: "For her conviction that America has a responsibility to halt or prevent the suffering of civilians abroad, she had been caricatured as the Ivy League Joan of Arc." Fueled by quotes from and about her, the characterization increasingly seems related to Power's voice, the act of her speaking. "I can't say anything that is not true," Power is quoted as saying, while about her, a fellow ambassador says, "She doesn't speak with flour in her mouth."

Because of the very providence or accident by which I was falling in the way of these occasions and the way they were speaking to me—always of language. Because what do we ask of language? How do we sort through what we will and will not say, what we can, what we can't?

Because I'm interested in the accidents of history and of our histories, how idiosyncratic—perhaps arbitrary—what we know, what we encounter, what we remember, what we miss, and the way brain chemistry, neurological state, is one kind of answer to these questions that are a theme of marvel and dismay in the daily conversation of my life.

Because every time I start with Joan, I start again at zero. Because don't we already know what we think about this?

Because perception, hallucination, and, it seems a safe bet, great pain.

Because, in some way, all of the above is refracted by or in my experience of migraines. And because sometimes, in the altered state that migraine imposes, I find myself acutely, at times even obsessively, interested in Joan—specifically, in her trial. That is, in what she had to say.

9

——

As usual, Anne Carson offers the most lucid distillation:

She was captured in battle on May 23, 1430. Her trial lasted from January to May of 1431 and entailed a magistrate's inquest, six public interrogations, nine private interrogations, an abjuration, a relapse, a relapse trial, and condemnation. Her death by fire took place on May 30, 1431. Thousands of words went back and forth between Joan and her judges during the months of her inquisition; many of them are available to us in some form.

The copiousness of the trial record was anomalous by design. Joan was an international celebrity at the time. The trial was political, ecclesiastical, social, historical, an actual battle in a real war. So the bishop charged with its execution (and, inevitably, with Joan's), asserting one kind of faith in language, made sure it was meticulously documented and that this documentation was assiduously copied, making it the most detailed and widely available trial record of the Middle Ages.

Among the fruits of these labors was the speed at which news of Joan's fate spread around the world. According to historian Daniel Hobbins, whose 2005 translation of the trial record is the one on which I rely, nine days after her death, notice was sent to "all the royalty of Europe" and later dispatches ensured that the story had become common knowledge across Western Europe by late summer. These labors also made it possible, twenty-five years after her death by fire, for a subsequent bishop to symbolically burn a copy of the original trial record on the occasion of its nullification. These labors also gave us Joan. "I don't know what you wish to ask me. Perhaps you might ask me things I can't tell you" are the first words we hear her say. Of course, she is far more often referred to than heard from.

a certain late woman, Joan

this woman utterly disregarding

this woman at the time

this woman so denounced

surrender the woman

this woman to us

this woman we ordered

this woman's words

the woman commonly called Joan the Maid

this woman was taken

this woman is hardly

the said Maid

this woman is

this woman to be handed over

bring the woman to this city

the said Joan

this Joan

(The article makes the object.)

Always a pack of them, the assembled masters for each hearing were carefully listed by name and station. The first public session consisted of forty-two men, including abbots, priors, doctors of theology, doctors of canon law, doctors of civil law, bachelors of theology, licentiates of canon and of civil law. Among them, thirteen Jeans interrogating one Jean d'Arc. The second public session: forty-eight, including abbots, priors, licentiates, a brother, a doctor of medicine, doctors of canon law, doctors of canon and civil law, fifteen doctors of theology, seven bachelors of theology, and two canons of Rouen; sixteen Jeans. Third session: sixty-one; fifteen.

asked her birthplace

asked the names

asked where

asked who

asked what

asked how

asked by

asked next

asked whether

asked whether

asked how

asked what

asked whether

asked what kind

asked whether

asked whether

(And so on.)

10

"In the interrogations," Hobbins notes of the Latin text, itself a translation of the French minutes recorded at the close of each day, "the verb tenses shift frequently from past to present." The sea of documents teems with damning accusations:

abandoned women's clothes; allowing herself to be adored; apostate; blasphemy; casting of spells; conjurer of evil spirits; contagion; corrupt member; credulous; cruel, cruel murders; cruelly thirsting; curses; dared to perform, to speak, and to publicize many things contrary; devilish malice; disregarding the honor due the female sex; disturber of the peace; divination; doubting; dressed and armed herself like a man; entangled in and practicing the magic arts; errors; evil-speaking; evil-thinking; false and deceitful; false heart; false prophetess; falsely imagined revelations; forgetting all feminine decency; hard-hearted; heresy; idolatry; incantations; inciting wars; incorrigible; invocation of demons; like a dog returning to its vomit; limb of Satan; maleficent; misdeeds; misled; moved by stubborn rashness; obstinate; offenses against the faith; other offenses; perjury of God's holy name; pernicious temptress; presumption; rash; rashly boasts; relapsed heretic; scandalous; schismatic; scornful; seditious; seduced and abused simple people; seduction of princes, nobles, clergy, and common people; seductress of princes and peoples; shocking and vile monstrosity; sorcery; spreading false dogmas; straying; superstition; throwing off the bridle of modesty; traffic with demons; transgressor; treason; unworthy of grace; usurping divine honor; various errors and wicked crimes

Most offensive to her accusers, even more than the audacity of claiming to hear voices sent directly from God, was her insistence on wearing men's clothes and, in them, assuming men's roles:

Wholly forsaking the decency and reserve of her sex, utterly without modesty and shamelessly having taken the disgraceful clothing and state of armed men . . .

But she absolutely refused and, as stated, steadfastly refuses to carry out other tasks proper to her sex, in all things behaving more like a man than a woman. With regard to this article, Joan says that she was in fact advised to wear women's clothes at Arras and in the castle of Beaurevoir; she refused then and still does. As for the other womanly tasks, she says there are enough other women to do them . . .

You took a short tunic, a doublet, and hose with many points; you wear your hair short, cut round above your ears, leaving nothing to indicate the female sex except what nature gave you. . . .

Most fascinating to us is her voice, what she will
and, especially, what she will not say:

> *"I took an oath for you yesterday; that should
> be quite enough for you."*

> *"You may well ask me some things that I will
> answer truthfully, and others that I will
> not."*

> *"Go on to the next question."*

> *"I will not tell you this."*

> *"I won't answer that."*

> *"What would you say if the voice has
> forbidden me?"*

> *"Believe me, it wasn't men who forbade me."*

> *"I'm not telling you all I know."*

> *"I request a delay."*

> *"You won't learn that yet."*

> *"I have nothing else to tell you."*

> *"You will get nothing more out of me on this."*

> *"Do you think you can catch me like this and
> draw me into your power?"*

"Even fire won't change my mind."

*"I have always told you that you will not
    drag that out of me. Go ask him,"*
    (meaning God).

And her voices:

She hears it many more times than she says.

*She answered that she was sleeping, and the
    voice woke her.*

She said it woke her without touching her.

The voice told her to answer boldly.

She never knew it to contradict itself.

*She said the light comes in the name of the
    voice.*

She recognizes them by their voices.

*She thinks she was around thirteen when the
    first voice came to her.*

*She said there was much light all around
    and this seemed fitting.*

She understood them perfectly.

In the end, we all know what happens. "Joan, dearest friend, now it is time at the end of your trial to think carefully about what has been said." Just prior to being condemned to death, Joan abjures and recants, agreeing to wear women's clothing and disavowing the voices. Reprieved or, rather, forgiven, instead of death she is given life, "a salutary penance of perpetual imprisonment, with the bread of sorrow and the water of affliction, that you may weep there for your faults." This on a Thursday.

By Friday or Saturday, she is back to wearing men's clothes. By Monday, she's insisting again that the voices are real. Tuesday, the council meets (thirty-nine, including three abbots, nine doctors of theology, two doctors of canon law, two archdeacons, five bachelors of theology, seven canons, eight licentiates, and a brother; ten Jeans). On Wednesday, she is condemned for heretical relapse in an expedited trial consisting of a public recitation of sins, then set ablaze before a crowd in the market square.

Moreover, we ourselves and certain learned and expert doctors and masters who were concerned for the salvation of your soul have often warned you on your behalf, duly and sufficiently, to correct and amend yourself in these matters. . . . Yet you would not do so, nor did you concern yourself with it, but in your hard-heartedness and stubbornness you positively denied the accusations and repeatedly refused to submit. . . .

11

It's remarkable how much primary knowledge we glean from the secondary arguments against it—a kind of negative proof—and from the procedural mechanisms intended to stamp it out. Joan's trial was nothing if not a procedure, an exercise in deep administration as a means of reining in a person deemed out of control. Of the hundreds upon hundreds of pages that make up the official record, Joan's words amount to only a small fraction. Epiphanic, resistant to standardization, full of lyric logic and lyric leaps, they are the swerving atoms, the collision-creations in an otherwise-sterile rain.

Constantly reasserting its own argument through persistent, plodding, painstakingly unoriginal form, procedure has a funny way of highlighting the very resistance it quashes. At least, within the confines of its dimly lit chambers, flashes of autonomy and originality seem to glimmer more brightly than just about anywhere else. Mapped onto body and mind, then, is the normal our procedural, a dull sky across which the abnormal flares? Such as inspiration? Such as pain?

The word *pain* derives from the Latin *poena* (penalty, punishment, execution), which itself derived from the ancient Greek *poine* (penalty, fine, blood money). Only later did notions of grief attach; later still, sensation. Here is the current order of meanings according to the *Oxford English Dictionary*:

1. *Suffering or loss inflicted as punishment for a crime or offence, a fine.*

2. *The state of or condition of consciousness arising from mental or physical suffering, an unpleasurable feeling or effect.*

3. *Bodily suffering, strongly unpleasant feeling in the body, such as arises from illness, injury, or harmful physical contact (a single sensation of this nature)*

(such sensations experienced during childbirth).

4. *Trouble taken in accomplishing or attempting something; careful and attentive effort.*

Is this the order you would have thought? This is not the order I would have thought. So much intermingling of category and implication of value, so many ghosts right there in front of us in the biography of the word.

"Ghosts may be grief gone awry," remarks Audrey Niffenegger, author of several collections of ghost stories, to explain their appeal. I'm not partial to ghost stories, but I love thinking about ghosts and grief in this way, and, more generally, about how one thing becomes another, especially by means of going awry.

For one thing, this is metaphor. And far from being frill on the surface of language, metaphor is fundamental to our ability to communicate, to know anything at all. For another thing, maybe this isn't metaphor. Alchemy, chemistry, translation, transformation, transmutation: one thing causes or becomes another (or seems to) around us, in us, all the time. Most compelling is the way these planes and processes inter-mingle and overlap: the figurative and the real, the mental and the physical, procedure and our resistance to it.

12

Kin to shows like *Murder, She Wrote*; *Law & Order*; and many others, *House M.D.* is a procedural, in this case medical. Every week, an impossible-to-solve case is solved (with occasional exceptions) by the mad-genius diagnostician Dr. Gregory House. The show employs many of the procedural's conventions, including establishing a recognizable and repetitive set of conventions.

Each episode begins with novel characters, unwitting patients-to-be whose symptoms, always dramatic, strike within ninety seconds. House, a cranky misanthrope, resists taking each case. Once taken, it's diagnosed via group brainstorm with his handpicked team of brilliant-in-their-own-right underling doctors who admire/loathe him and via batteries of tests they run to narrow down their hypotheses. A cheesy trope of the camera entering the patient's body for an edifying microscopic journey is deployed. Inevitably, several wrong diagnoses are pursued before the right one is landed upon, or, more accurately, revealed. It's always when House goes to buy a sandwich, gratuitously badger a colleague, or minister to an uninteresting clinic patient that he has his breakthrough. Along the way, ethical limits are stretched, personal boundaries are breached. Okay, fine.

Like most good serials and more than many decent procedurals, beneath the surface content the show is about the characters' relationships with one another and to themselves—their hopes and fears, their pasts, their limits. At the center is House, who, in addition to being a diagnostic genius, lives with acute pain stemming from a misdiagnosed blood clot in his femoral artery that led to muscle death, disfigurement, and a pronounced limp. He is also addicted to pain pills. As a result, within the reassuring structures of a predictable procedural playground fueled by medical mystery gotchas, more than anything else the show is about pain, the acute, chronic variety: its experience, its consequences, its refusal to resolve.

Premise: Body dysfunction is unpredictable, complex, a cascading effect, a runaway train to be stopped, a mystery to be solved.

Premise: Body function is mappable, knowable, organized and orderly, but only to a certain extent. Like a medieval map, the known world of the body has outer reaches, beyond which there is a vast sea full of monsters that fades to black: the unknown world of the body.

Premise: We are wrong many times before we are right.

Premise: Which is better/which is worse: the solvable unknown or the unsolvable known? Hint, House's original affliction was curable but unknown and therefore uncured; now it is known but incurable and he devotes his life to transforming unknowns into knowns. (Hope rubs both ways.)

Premise: When we grasp for it, the key we are searching for remains out of reach. Epiphanic revelation (a form of mental creation) most often comes through distraction, slant association, accidental juxtaposition—that is to say, swerve.

13

Let's go further back. It is remarkable how much primary knowledge we glean from the secondary arguments against it, much like the way House throws meds at a failing patient in order to rule out certain conditions when they don't work or when they wreak a signature kind of havoc.

Antiphon the Sophist was a late-fifth-century B.C. philosopher, rhetorician, and interpreter of dreams. In addition to working as a teacher and a speechwriter for the court, he was a purveyor of "verbal medicine," for which he was ridiculed by the comic-philosophers (who knew?) of his day. Apparently, alongside politics and money, Antiphon was interested in dismantling superstitions, advising that people should not be afraid of dreams or put much stock in divination, both widely used diagnostic methods of his day. He was interested, too, in pain; more specifically, in dodging it: among his works are believed to have been a treatise titled *The Art of Freedom from Pain* and a manual called *Avoidance of Grief.*

As is common to many of his era, all we have left of Antiphon are fragments of his work and, more expansively, later references to—mostly arguments against—it. Perhaps this is for the best. He is believed to have advertised lessons in painlessness and claimed that "no one could tell him a sorrow so terrible that he could not remove it from the teller's mind."

Ranging from single words to the occasional suite of full paragraphs, 118 fragments survive. Collected in Katherine Freeman's 1948 *Ancilla to the Pre-Socratic Philosophers* (a complete translation of the fifth edition of Hermann Diels's *Fragamente der Vorsokratiker*), the text occasionally coheres into extended arguments, only to quickly disintegrate again into strange, often beautiful word islands that, stacked together, form numinous lists.

Shadowfeet

Longheads

Dwellers underground

Sometimes no primary text—not even a word—
survives, but secondary ghosts of reference and
inference remain. Whenever possible, Freeman provides context within which to situate
the remnant text's fractured, or even missing,
utterances, noting what larger work they're
thought to survive or what argument they
might have been asserting. In this spirit, she
frequently makes note of Antiphon's "unusual"
word choices, and quite often these remarkable usages relate to perception that, in keeping
with established pre-Socratic tradition, he links
directly to pain. Such a focus makes sense: for
a mind interested in the ground of perception
(experience) as pain (to be avoided), the words
used to describe it are gates that swing wide or
slam shut to determine the very field.

*(Word for "unseen" used to mean "things not
seen but thought to be seen")*

(Word for "unfelt" used to mean "things not felt but thought to be felt")

(Words for "look through" and "visible")

(Words for "sight")

(Words for "smell")

When therefore in the air there occurs a clash of contrary winds and showers.

(Word for "gone over again from the beginning")

(Word for "proceed")

("Exchanges" used for "combinations" or "mixings")

(Word for "the prevailing arrangement of the Whole")

(Word for "that which is still unarranged")

By an eddy

(To give an analgesic for headache): To stupefy

(Word for): having blood

Not to be seen

Bivouacking (for "sleeping")

Manageable (metaphor from driving horses)

Doubling and halving

Cuttle-fish (signifies escape)

14

Antiphon was preceded in his focus on pain by Anaxagoras and other pre-Socratic philosophers who proposed that existence equals perception and perception equals pain (pleasure equals pain followed close behind). In "Anaxagoras on Perception, Pleasure, and Pain," James Warren offers a sort of CliffsNotes:

(1) *The like is unaffected by the like.*

(2) *(Perception is or involves an affection.) [Implicit]*

(3) *Therefore all perception occurs via opposites.*

(4) *Every unlike with which we come into contact causes exertion/toil.*

(5)   *Therefore all perception involves exertion/toil.*

(6)   *(Toil is painful.) [Implicit]*

(7)   *Therefore all perception involves pain.*

Arguing against Anaxagoras's position, rival philosopher Theophrastus describes it more vividly: "[He says that] every perception is accompanied by pain. . . . For every unlike we contact causes distress. . . . For bright colors and excessively loud noises produce pain and we are unable to withstand the same ones for very long."

Anaxagoras may have been laying foundation for the larger house of embodied experience, but like Antiphon's fragments, his postulations render a kind of migraine diagram. That is, through the lens of migraine, these formulations become descriptive, immediate, encompassing. Here, as elsewhere, migraine takes an abstraction and makes it concrete. And apparently Anaxagoras believed that perception—inherently painful, as established—was centered in the head.

The subsequent unspooling of pre-Socratic philosophy pertaining to the compresence of pain and pleasure is one that I resist, so I'm glad it doesn't speak to the subject at hand, except insofar as the way acute pain allows for acute awareness of lack of pain when it resolves—a strange and private kind of pleasure, a hallowed hall into which one steps, like the stately space of silence after prolonged noise, or anything, really, that allows us to perceive absence as physically manifest.

"After great pain, a formal feeling comes" is how, more than two thousand years after Anaxagoras, Emily Dickinson put it. "Horse, then, unhorses what is not horse," offered C. D. Wright approximately 150 years later, speaking to the power of language—itself a form of perception based on collision-creation—to make and unmake by naming, but also to the invention-interplay between states of being.

What am I trying to get at in the arrangement of these postulations chipped from the columns of the past? Existence is perception and perception is pain and this is a road map to what? I'm not here interested in the premise, more concisely laid

out in Buddhist tracts, that all life is suffering—
not because it's inaccurate, not because it's equal
parts delightful and disconcerting to see founda-
tional precepts of Eastern and Western philosophy overlap, not because here we have yet another
example of Western culture's pervasive habit of
sticking a flag into already well-established ideas
or practices and declaring them discovered, but
because it feels so dismayingly inert.

Rather, I'm interested in collisions, in accidents,
in the idea that this is how things spring into
being and how we are made of that: all things
born of disorderly action. Perception is our ability—our imperative—to experience with our
bodies this action of which our bodies themselves and everything around them are com-
posed. This experiencing is a form of pain. Pain
beyond the level of this baseline, migraine with
its acute pain and heightened perception, then,
is a vividly colored, volume-turned-way-up version of just this, of our fundamental nature and
environment, of reality. So is dealing with it.

"One need not be a Chamber—to be Haunted
. . ." (Dickinson again).

15

"Oh, I wish we still thought it was that, that was easy to explain," sighs my neurologist when I ask her for migraine's most current definition—if it's still based on vasoconstriction—a question I ask every few years so as to track, but not too closely, the ever-changing science. She's sitting in a lab coat on a wheeled office chair, my chart in her hand, and on the stainless-steel table in front of her, the dozen or so needles she's just used to inject precisely titrated doses of Onabotchulinum toxin A into my face and scalp, each one a wasp sting. It's important that she count the needles again before disposing of them in the Sharps container; this is a rigorously controlled procedure.

"We used to think it was the blood vessels in the brain narrowing or dilating or spasming.

That was something people could picture. Now, at least according to the last conference I went to, they think it's an at least sixteen-phase neurological cascade ranging all the way from the brain stem to the prefrontal cortex. To be honest," she continues, "I didn't really understand it. I could tell you more if I had the handout in front of me—there were some beautiful charts and images—I'll see if I can find it for you."

It took me years to try Botox ("for migraine," I always feel compelled to say). Because it's expensive and was initially somewhat controversial, and also because it works only on very specific kinds of headaches, you have to jump through a significant number of hoops before you can be approved for treatment: careful documentation of the right kind of migraines and the right kind of failed attempts to treat them with the right kind of medications over the right length of time. I'd run the requisite course many times over, for years had been an "eligible candidate," but I shied away, uncertain about the results studies were showing and worried about potentially terrifying, albeit very rare, side effects unable to be reversed simply by stopping a given pill. They say the medicine—a strong neurotoxin—is effective for three months, but accounting for its half-life, each dose haunts the body for considerably longer.

Our cures are as many as they are elusive. Long have we needed them, long have we searched for them, our fickle, beloved cures. And how to judge if they're working? Taking up the vast space between miraculous good and hideous harm is the land of not quite being sure. I mean, maybe they're better. This month, I think, was better. Or, this month was bad, but who knows how bad it would have been without [fill-in-the-blank]?

Sourcing widely, perhaps wildly, from his own far-flung travels, the august texts of his day, and deep wells of local folklore, Pliny the Elder—a first-century A.D. Roman naturalist, author, and naval commander—cataloged seemingly all the available knowledge of his day. Ranging from astronomy to the nature of man and war to flora and fauna the world over, his *Natural History* includes a panoply of both ailments and cures.

Himself a sufferer, Pliny mentions asthma only once in his magnum opus, at least according to the Penguin edition currently available—"Vinegar checks chronic coughs, catarrh of the throat, asthma, and shrinkage of the gums"—despite its looming large in his own life. Whether foolishly indulging his curiosity or only having gone there in hopes of rescuing a friend, Pliny died in Pompeii during the eruption of Vesuvius, when toxic fumes overcame his weak lungs. (His crew, whom he had instructed to tie pillows to their heads as protection from falling pumice, survived.)

Six entries address headache. Who doesn't get them: "inhabitants of India or Ethiopia who stand over seven feet tall, never spit, and never suffer headache, toothache, or pain in the eyes." What helps cure them: "raw cabbage in the morning combined with several other ingredients; a garland of pennyroyal" (which also protects the head from injury, cold, heat, and thirst); "a band of thalassaegle around the head; cutting the hair on the 17th and 29th of the month"; and this:

> *People say that if one pares a corn when a star is falling, it is very quickly cured, and one can relieve a pain in the head by applying a poultice from vinegar poured over door-hinges.*

Similarly, a rope used by someone who has hanged himself relieves headaches if tied round the temples.

After two and a half years of expensive injections every three months, painful during and for a few days after, I'm still not sure if it's helping. Maybe? Like many treatments, Botox as migraine therapy was discovered accidentally. A subset of people, mostly women, getting cosmetic injections to smooth facial wrinkles experienced a decrease in the number of headaches they suffered. Enough of them noticed, and bothered to say something, and eventually, one supposes, were believed, for the anecdotal to cohere into studies and protocols. Today's therapeutic treatment is distinct from the cosmetic procedure in strain, dose, strength, and placement, but was from it accident-born. A kind of selection for coincidental side effect, unintended and ill understood, but hey, nothing else works, so let's try it—just like betablockers, SSRIs, tricyclics, hormone-replacement therapies, antiseizure medications, and many more.

Premises:

"And if we're wrong?" "We learn something else."

"You know, there are other ways to manage pain." "Like what? Laughter, meditation? You got a guy who can fix my third chakra?"

"Pills don't make me high; they make me neutral."

"You're cranky." "I'm in pain."

"So, what does the pain tell us? It tells us nothing." (*House M.D.*)

Medications and Alternative Therapies Tried (partial list):

acupuncture, betablockers, bioidentical hormones, birth-control pills, Botox, butterbur, calcium/magnesium supplements, calcium channel blockers, chelation, chi gung, Chinese herbs, chiropractic adjustment, cranial-sacral manipulation, cupping, hormone-replacement therapy, Depakote, Elavil, elimination diet, Estradiol, feverfew, Fioricet, fish oil, Florinef, Frova, gluten- corn- caffeine- alcohol-free diets, gua sha, homeopathy,

Imitrex, massage, Maxalt, meditation, megadose vitamin IVs, Naratriptan, Neurontin, nonsteroidal anti-inflammatories (multiple), nortriptlyine, ondansetron, osteopathic manipulation, Paxil, physical therapy, reiki, Relpax, rotation diet, Seasonique, tai chi, Topamax, trigger-point injections, tui na, wild yam cream, yoga.

Side Effects Experienced (partial list):

Brain fog, constipation, depression, diarrhea, difficulty concentrating, dissociation, dizziness, fatigue, hypotension, inability to find words, increased headaches, irritability, lethargy, memory loss, mental changes (other), mood changes (other), muscle weakness, nausea, numbness, sexual problems, skin sensitivity, stuttering, sweating, tingling, tremor, twitching, weight gain, weight loss, withdrawal.

"Isn't there anything they can *do*?" my father (a doctor) asks at the end of the conversation about how my headaches are, which we have almost every time he calls.

16

All good theories are falsifiable. In me. By me. But which? When? How? So consistent in their assertions and yet so unpredictable in how they act, meaning react—to medication, to the movements of the day—it's hard to know what I'm in for with any given migraine. "Sometimes I wake up with the pain at a five," I say, resorting to the kind of scale I hate, "take one pill and I'm fine for the day. Other times I wake up at a five and three pills later it's like I haven't taken anything." "Yeah," says my neurologist sympathetically. "We don't understand that. It probably depends on where you happen to be in the cascade."

We operate always within the blinkered confines of our current knowledge, a fish-eyed sphere of walled-off vision that reveals no walls until we bump up against them, and even then, not always. Just recognizing the limitations of our view is often tremendously hard-won, but it's of limited use: even when we apprehend its outer edges, we can't see beyond them—we can barely imagine the boundary line shifting, let alone the wall budging loose.

I was four in the summer of 1976, when Bob Seger's "Night Moves" began its long run as a mainstay on FM radio.

> *I was a little too tall*
>
> *Could've used a few pounds*
>
> *Tight pants points hardly renown*
>
> *She was a black-haired beauty with big dark*
> *   eyes*
>
> *And points all her own sitting way up high*
>
> *Way up firm and high . . .*

Loving it from a preadolescent age, I was too young to comprehend the sexual nature of the lyrics, so I understood the teenage pair not as lovers, but as budding private eyes sneaking off to practice their, you know, investigation stuff.

*Out past the cornfields where the woods got
   heavy*

Out in the back seat of my '60 Chevy

Workin' on mysteries without any clues

Workin' on our night moves . . .

Into the void created by my inability to read the data, I projected a version of it seamlessly transformed into something readable at just my level. Mishearing occurs in the ear but also in the mind.

Misseeing is even more abstruse. A feature of binocular vision is that each eye has a blind spot and together they compensate for this weakness. Collating input from two optic nerves, the brain fills in the empty space, hiding absence by projecting the known onto the unknown. Which is to say, we don't know what we don't see, literally. Through similar mechanisms, without testing designed to isolate each eye, certain degenerative diseases can progress unchecked for a long time: a defect in the peripheral field often grows to be enormous before we perceive its presence. And when it does, when we do, it's never by looking at something straight on. We learn of our deficit by what blindsides us, what hits us, seemingly, from out of nowhere.

Example (good): "Have you found anything that increases the pain?" this massage therapist asks, going over my intake form. My ear stutter-steps, almost hearing the more typical question, the one I expect her to ask, something along the lines of "Have you found anything that decreases it?" How unusual: instead of rushing in—good intentions, hubris, and blind spots in tow—to see how she can make it better, she wants first to see how she can make it not worse.

Example (bad): This doctor believes he understands my "very serious condition" and is sure he has the cure. When my symptoms don't respond to his protocol, he tells me he's no longer convinced my "general feeling of malaise" has any underlying cause at all.

Example (bad): This holistic practitioner, frustrated by an increase in migraines coinciding with her care, looks meaningfully into my eyes and says, "You're going to have to find another way of expressing yourself."

Example (typical): This Pilates instructor interrupts our stretching to show me a reflexology point on my big toe. Digging into it mercilessly, she says this is how she aborts her own headaches, no matter how bad, and now she never gets them. Dutifully, I dig, and keep trying all week to see if this might be my stumbled-upon miracle, too. She's visibly disappointed when I report back miracleless.

Example (from the literature): This esteemed physician, in the foreword to another esteemed physician's book on migraine, offers an insider's point of view: "Because of the lack of full comprehension of the complexities and variabilities of a condition which is in every way fascinating in its phenomenology, many doctors are only too pleased when a patient, in desperation, takes himself off to practitioners of 'fringe medicine,' almost hoping that the results will be both disastrous and very costly." (William Gooddy)

Example (horse's mouth): "Nothing is more threatening to who you think you are than a patient with a problem you cannot solve." (Atul Gawande)

Conclusion (one of many): It's not only our own hope and fear that treacherously we navigate; it's lots of other people's, too.

17

On the Saturday soccer field, the six- to eight-year-olds are dropping like flies. Many team sports incorporate the art of the flop—a strategically exaggerated response to physical contact—as one among a handful of commonly played mind games pertaining to health and strength, but none quite as integrally as soccer. Spanish is the common language at the Eastside Y, but we don't speak it, and this makes the drop and roll, the dry-grass writhing harder to read.

Pain as autonomic reaction or pain as performance? Pain performed as advantage, seduction, evidence wholly forged or simply highlighted for easier viewing? Something happened or I want you to believe it did. Here, see it, let me help you. The act makes visible the invisible or invented, broadcasts what otherwise might remain private.

"What'd you do?" a colleague asks with a smile when he sees me cantilevering down the hall in a postsurgical boot. Over the course of several years, he's barely spoken to me, has never inquired about anything, really. Something about the visible sign that points to pain, but in a fun athletic injury or human foible kind of way, invites comment, opens the door. My answer, toe surgery for a congenital defect, leaves nowhere amusing for the conversation to go, so it ends. Given the opportunity, we'd rather not look at all. Compelled or invited to look, we quickly invite ourselves to look away.

The interaction brings to mind another from some years back with another usually reticent male colleague. "When are you due?" he blurted out with an unmediated mix of incredulity, revulsion, and alarm upon seeing me eight months pregnant, and lumbering up the stairs. For some conditions, there's no possibility of flopping. Invisibility has its price, but visibility does, too.

Once over a period of weeks, I invented a serial story for my son about a misfit band of underwater friends—an orphaned mermaid, an octopus into decorating, an immature beluga whale, and an implacable old turtle—who lived in the unhaunted part of the mermaid's castle left to her by her father. Every morning, they breakfasted on food natural to their kind but repulsive to one other. By appointment each month, they visited the mermaid's sister at the edge of a certain dock, both parties having traveled several days to get there, the underwater crew by sea, the no-longer-mermaid sister by land—years ago she had given up her tail for love of birdsong and forest. (She didn't regret her decision, but she did miss swimming, which, according to the bargain she had struck, was now forbidden.)

The gang's other adventures came by way of a treasure map leading them to secret alcoves within the ocean—kelp forest, whirlpool, birthplace of bubbles, source of darkness, origin of light—where its magical powers were stored. They also visited the beluga's mother, who missed him. One day, compelled to face the fear they lived with, they unlocked the scariest room in the haunted part of the castle and found there a tortured zombie-shark swimming in circles and thirsting for blood. I don't remember why I stopped telling the story.

Actually, I do. Over time, it became formulaic, almost procedural. I grew tired of it, I grew bored, so I'd take longer and longer breaks between installments, and then I'd forget where we'd left off, how we might begin again. I barely remember any of it now. Margo was the mermaid's name, the one who still lived in the sea. A reminder of how much passes through us, sheds off us, the fleeting nature of processes such as parenthood, such as pain? Two weeks into my time away, with much fanfare after only brief daily phone calls, I Skype with my son to tell him a bedtime story. Looking at each other, we both end up sad. It made a pain visible. Or, visible, we made a pain. Neither was helpful.

18

Postulation:

"I'm not saying you're not in pain."

"You're saying my pain is a cliché."

"I'm saying pain fades."

"Did yours?"

"Physical pain is different."

"I'd rather have my leg chopped off—"

"You don't know that because you haven't felt—"

"Neither have you." (*House M.D.*)

Thought experiment is a dignified name for a frequently desperate process: *What if? What if? What if?* Not only the constant weighing of potential courses of action, their pros and cons, not only the necessary guesswork of what will be possible, reasonable—*Can I stand up? Can I drive? Can I work today? How long before I'm able? Then, for how long will I be able?*—but the magical thinking, too, the make-believe bargaining you can't help but do. More than anything, it's a means of proving yourself to you, rehearsing how much you don't want this to be happening.

Would I cut off a hand? Yes, the left. *Quit my dream job?* As long as we had enough to eat. *Give up having had my first love?* Don't ask me that. Maybe. I guess so. *Let harm come to my child?* No. *Give up poetry?*

"That's good. That's unusual," muttered my most trusted doctor years ago, seemingly to herself after testing the strength of my grip while I repeated certain phrases: *I want to be healthy. I want to be sick. I want to be completely healthy. I want to be a little bit sick.* In the hands of someone less expert, less compassionate, I would have refused. "No part of you seems to be identifying with your condition," she said briskly, "which is, for the most part, good. Frequently in long-term patients we see an identification develop that is important to address."

Sympathy likes a crisis: novelty, drama, limited duration, potential for heroics. Around a crisis, community springs up heartfelt and energetic, but time-limited—its crest is the beginning of its drop. Crisis passes and so do the pop-up structures it supports. It's probably evolutionary: chronic tends to bore us, all that persistent, unchanging need. Plus, crises arrive, demanding our attention! One way or another, when it comes to chronic, most of us reach the outer limits of empathy's gravitational pull and then slip right on through. What, then, to do with a condition that is both: crisis and chronic, a kind of emergency set on endless, if intermittent and variable, repeat?

"I would take it from you if I could," my mother says over the phone, regularly.

When the days pile up, I start thinking about being dead—not suicide, really, a fantasy instead: the pleasure of waking into a kind of bodilessness, which is sometimes how the clearing (*that formal feeling*) feels when it finally does come. On the one hand, pain is isolating, makes you an island, makes you distant, makes you selfish, unable to spare your energy or even your concern. On the other hand, it removes your armor, makes you vulnerable, shrinks distances, makes you more connected, more permeable than ever before. In pain, certain kinds of separation materialize, but others fall away. The thick glass walls of health invisibly buffering body and mind crack or, somehow, dissolve.

The homeless person begging change at the already-cacophonous intersection is one of many things too many in the fraying state of worsening migraine, but there is also a slide inside the pain, and without choosing to, without thinking about it at all, I imagine her pain from within the shatter of my own, which is already intolerable, even properly fed and cleanly clothed and fully housed, even well cared for. I project onto her my pain in her situation, and though this is false—though I know I know nothing of who she is, how she feels, what she endures—in this way, in all its mistakenness, I imagine her. There is no wall. Instead, I'm everywhere skirting ledges over which things might calamitously fall.

Some ways of being alive are worse than not living—on this, don't we all agree? I'm not guess-
ing into the panhandler now, I'm talking about
myself. It has always seemed obvious that without medication to control it, the pain would be
too much. Mostly, I imagine stepping from a
roof; I'm not sure why. Maybe because it'd be
breezy up there and sometimes a breath of cool,
fresh air can provide a moment of relief from
migraine's hot, pressing hand. Maybe because
the roof is the head of the body of the building.

This isn't suicidal ideation and I'm not
depressed. It's executive function functioning,
a barely sketched strategic plan—only a little,
just a hazy understanding with myself because
I am one of the lucky unlucky; I am not without medication, and mostly the medication does
work. Eventually, it works. Still, I notice an
anxiety while driving Texas highways that I've
never felt before. I'm not afraid of Boston's narrow, overtrafficked streets teeming with aggressive drivers. I've driven happily in Manhattan,
San Francisco, Athens. But Austin's interstates
terrify me a little in their sweeping expanses
flung out to the sky. Something is off in the

color of the asphalt, in the angle of the sun, but mostly it's the towering overpasses, over which you see only blue: the rickety roofs they imply.

19

_____

Angor animi: fear for the soul, sense of imminent dissolution

Cephalalgia: head pain, nothing more

I'm not sick. I'm in pain. I'm not searching for meaning in it, because it doesn't mean anything. "People get what they get. It has nothing to do with what they deserve," House snaps in response to a sentimental comment. I'm not saying life is meaningless in general or that mine lacks meaning in particular. I'm saying there's no *there* there, or, only there is *there*. I'm saying, lady, would you say that to a five-year-old wasting away on the cancer ward? Do you think the dying elm just needs to say something about its days as a sapling? Don't you believe in biology anymore?

*Sometimes it's like someone took a knife,
    baby, edgy and dull*

*And cut a six-inch valley through the middle
    of my skull*

*At night I wake up with the sheets soaking
    wet*

*And a freight train running through
    the middle of my head . . .*
    (Bruce Springsteen)

The song may claim to be about desire, but in these lines at least, I'm not buying it, Bruce — that's pain. Greedy, gaudy, god-awful, this often overwhelming feature of existence, of my existence—it just *is*, it just *does*, it doesn't *mean*. Which isn't to say there's not plenty to learn.

Lesson (season 1, episode 11, "Detox"): Transitive Properties, or, to Focus Is to Erase

Off Vicodin on a bet, House's pain (a combination of original injury and withdrawal symptoms) becomes overwhelming. Desperate to make it stop, he delivers a vicious blow to his left hand using a clublike pestle from a decorative apothecary set. First he grimaces; then he grins; then he leans back in an effluence of relief. "The brain has a gating mechanism for pain, registers the most severe injury and blocks out the others," he explains a few minutes later to the friend splinting his broken hand. "Did it work?" his friend asks. "Well, my hand hurts like hell. Yeah, I feel much better," House replies before requesting a soft splint in case he needs to rattle the gate again.

See also: "One's character must necessarily grow like that with which one spends the greater part of the day." (Antiphon, 62)

Lesson (season 3, episode 13, "Insensitive"): Silence Speaks Its Own Language

Fascinated by a patient with a rare genetic disorder that results in a total inability to perceive pain, House grows increasingly desperate in his desire to decode her brain's language of unsaying. Hounded as he is, she represents a kind of living holy grail. She won't play along, though—not only regarding his interest but also with respect to his assumption—arguing the pain of lack of pain, the injuries she's endured without realizing or unwittingly self-inflicted, the crippling nature of her daily self-care and precautionary limitations. They end up in a petulant debate, trying to one-up each other's suffering at the hands of opposite conditions—ever pain/ never pain—each railing against his or her own version of imprisonment, refusing to acknowledge the paradoxical similarity of their respective cells.

See also: "Justice, then, is not to transgress that which is the law of the city in which one is a citizen." (Antiphon, 44)

Lesson (season 5, episode 12, "Painless"): Careful What You Wish For

Working on the case of a man suffering from such acute chronic pain that he repeatedly tries to kill himself (including while in the hospital, with the help of his young son), House and his team explore a wide range of potential causes. Among the possibilities considered is opioid-induced hyperalgesia: pain caused by the very medications used to treat it. They postulate that while the patient's pain may have originated due to some other cause, it has long since evolved into a treatment-fulfilling prophecy. "Pain and the drugs that treat pain work by changing brain chemistry, sometimes to the point where brain receptors read painkillers as killer pain," House explains. In order to test the hypothesis, they put the patient through the agony of abruptly stopping his pain meds: if the pain is opioid-induced, after an excruciating withdrawal, the body's pain receptors should reset. They don't; they can't; the team was wrong—in this case, that was not the cause, so pain cannot treat the pain the patient is in.

See also: "Nothing, however hot, could not be hotter." (Anaxagoras)

Lesson (season 5, episode 15, "Softer Side"): You Are What You Eat

This one is different. No backstory, no lead-up. One day, House is acting nice. He humors a patient's worried parents by pursuing an unnecessary test; he chooses not to torment a colleague when given the opportunity; he treats clinic patients kindly. It turns out he's traded in his Vicodin for methadone and, although dangerous (at one point it causes him to stop breathing), it takes his pain away. For this, he's willing to risk serious harm, even death, but also, at his friends' urging, to take great care: he hires someone to monitor his breathing while he sleeps; he agrees to a carefully supervised regimen. Before his boss/friend/love interest accepts his new treatment protocol, he's even willing to leave his job, supposedly the most important thing in his otherwise-pain-stunted life. But then he misses a diagnosis. Fueled by lack-of-pain-induced ease or absence of dis-ease, he makes different decisions or he makes decisions differently: the case gets confused and he fails to solve a mystery he ordinarily would have cracked. The patient ends up fine; the problem is not one of guilt. The problem is that without the irritation of his pain, that toil, without its friction, its urgency, something—it's hard to say exactly what—he isn't himself. His genius is linked to his pain, and without it, his genius diminishes. So he stops taking the methadone.

See also: "Eclipses of the moon are caused by the turning of its bowl." (Antiphon, 28)

20

The procedural is a form, and form itself is a
kind of language. Occasional story lines not-
withstanding, mostly *House M.D.* speaks to
pain through the repeated syntax of the episodes' unfolding. Direct, even strenuously up
front about House's condition—the pain and
the pills—every installment articulates him living with both, repeating certain moves to make
sure we know it. Never far from reach and frequently renewed, the prescription pill bottle
is ever in pocket, in hand, perched on bathtub
ledge or nightstand. Regularly, House throws
back several Vicodin at a time like a practiced
pro: straight, no chaser. Not infrequently,
we see him wince or, when no one's looking,
unmask a deeper expression of anguish, mas-
saging his mutilated thigh. As constant as the

actor's American accent (Hugh Laurie is English), his pronounced limp and cane dependence
never falter.

A more provocative means of foregrounding
House's pain is the frequency with which his
friends (a complicated designation) and peers
(likewise) mention it—not seriously, although
from time to time they do that, too, but flip-
pantly, in the style of verbal joust. A characteristic interaction looks like this: When
he acquiesces unusually easily to a new case,
House's boss/friend/love interest says, "That
was easy." He responds, "We're in an elevator, I
can't exactly run away." To which she responds,
eyebrows raised, "It's not like you can run away
anyway." "Ouch," he replies, mock-hurt, "that's
just mean."

Bits like this, what do they signify? Maybe the
show is just trying to be edgy. Maybe his friends
are mirroring back to House the kind of jokes
he makes about himself or his tendency toward
bluntness, even cruelty. But something more
seems at stake. The bullying is acceptable—
playful, flirtatious even—because House is the

one in charge: he's the real bully, and his excuse, as much as his genius, is his pain. In mocking him, they're actually mocking it. The jokes highlight their own superficiality: they work to distinguish House's pain from House himself; they assert that his condition is insignificant, even tangential, to the exceptional whole of who he is. It is House who argues the opposite, insisting that his pain is inseparable from him and so, too, his need to treat it.

Does our pain define us? Only if it's bad enough? Only if we let it? Only if we don't have anything else going on? Because he's brilliant, the jibes seem to say, House's pain need not define him. But House's pain largely does define him. It's pervasive, he's never free of it, it reaches into every part of his life. Is this disconnect, then, what is meant to be revealed—an incommunicableness, an untranslatability at the core?

"There are two kinds of silence that trouble a translator: physical, metaphysical," Anne Carson writes. Here, the physical silence of which she speaks is external, the vacuum that surrounds an ancient fragment separated from whatever company it once kept. Metaphyiscal silence, on the other hand, "is silence that happens inside words themselves." Referring to the difficulty of moving between tongues, she could as easily be describing the language of pain: "Every translator knows the point where one language cannot be rendered into another." The problem isn't a superficial one concerning definitions or usage; rather, it runs almost unfathomably deep. "What if, within this silence, you discover a deeper one—a word that does not intend to be translatable? A word that stops itself." Here she turns by way of Homer to a language "known only to the gods." From there she turns to Joan.

21

"With its stunning camerawork and striking compositions, Carl Theodor Dreyer's *The Passion of Joan of Arc* convinced the world that movies could be art," declaims the Criterion Collection's introductory gloss. The much-lauded film devoted to Joan's ordeal went through ordeals of its own. Censored, destroyed by fire, painstakingly restored, destroyed by fire again, for more than fifty years it survived only in mutilated, bastardized form. "Then, in 1981, an original Danish copy, complete and in very good condition, was miraculously discovered in a closet of a Norwegian mental institution." The reconstituted French version of this copy resulted in a film considered to be "probably very close to the original."

After months of waiting for just the right moment, finally I watch it. I understand that it was shot in 1928. I understand that nearly everything about our understanding of cinema and acting and women was different then. I understand, too, that silent movies must find alternative ways to speak. Shot by shot, I find the film beautiful: lush of tone, masterfully framed. But I hate it. This Joan—wide-eyed and quivering, weepy and girlish, dreamy and vague, a nightmare, really, of male-gaze-defined feminine virtue in all its fainting, feinting, by gosh a little wispy bit of gumption—this Joan is no Joan of mine.

I find myself fascinated, though, by how more than three-quarters of the way through the film, in the scenes depicting Joan's conviction for relapse and her subsequent execution, Dreyfus seems to step before our very eyes from the realm of photography into the realm of film. For eighty-seven minutes we've inhabited a visual world overwhelmingly made up of closely held, wildly carved human faces that process across the screen like a series of richly toned black-and-white portraits reminiscent not only of still photography but of Renaissance paintings, Byzantine icons, even Greek and Roman busts. The effect is so pervasive that when these living faces move, they look like objects put through the motions of stop-action animation.

Then, suddenly, Dreyfus gives us the outdoors, where before we had been exclusively inside; he gives us commoners, where before we had only clergy and duncelike dungeon staff, and among these commoners are women, and we realize we've been in a world made up exclusively of men plus Joan: Joan of men's clothes and close-cropped hair, Joan of highly stylized near-hysterical wide-eyed ecstasy and fear, of erotically infused enthusiasm and cloyingly "feminine" tears, circled, always circled, by statues-come-to-life men, a parade of them usually, pouring into the frame as if clown-car sprung.

But now we have smoke from the fire that will kill and a crowd—messy folk with their mushy faces and missing teeth, their stupid caps, their base bloodlust, and their soft-spined sorrow—all of them quick-cut, blurry, chaotic. And then in the midst of it, clear and steady, the camera closes in on an infant suckling. No woman whole, just breast and baby. The infant pauses in its work, comes off the nipple—ostensibly to stare for an unbearably "pregnant" moment at the stage on which the pageant of Joan's death is playing out—then returns to it, latching good, sucking hard.

The baby is a blunt stroke, a silly gesture, but what haunts the screen is the exposed nipple: unblocked, unblurred, fully erect, for a brief moment a truer subject of the camera's and, through it, the viewer's gaze. After so much strenuous reaching after *meaning*, after so much gendered hash, the expressionless, naked nipple—simply and mutely there—comes as an unexpected relief. It may be the only honest shot, the only honest utterance, in the whole affair.

22

Early in *The Body in Pain*, Elaine Scarry identifies pain (of the acute physical variety) as fundamentally inexpressible in language: "Physical pain has no voice. . . . Its resistance to language is not simply one of its incidental attributes but is essential to what it is." In the grips of it, she says, we don't exactly go mute; we go prelanguage—reduced or returned to a state of utterance that is literally moan and groan. "Physical pain does not simply resist language but actively destroys it, bringing about an immediate reversion to a state anterior to language, to the sounds and cries a human being makes before language is learned." Less your island is vanishing into the sea and more you're the island that's vanishing.

Setting off from this port, Scarry promises to explore "why pain should require this shattering of language," but I find myself wanting to linger here, in the shatter. What if alongside destruction is creation? Aren't shards the material of mosaics? That is, what if instead of prelanguage, pain is extralanguage: outside of the norms by which dominant modes of language typically order and mean? Might this outsideness encompass resistance (genius-rage) and untranslatability (unbridgeable divide), alongside the possibility—even the necessity—of invention?

The trouble with standard pain scales, it seems to me, is that they weren't written by the right people—the people in pain. Often misheard as language that does not communicate, it turns out that the seemingly chaotic fragments of description people in pain manage to offer in fact cohere into meaningful systems of categorization. Researchers, Scarry tells us, have gathered up the shards and found logic in their arrangement, mapping dimensions relevant not only to diagnosis but also to treatment and sometimes even cure.

Throbbing, flickering, quivering, pulsing, beating: temporal dimension

Burning, hot, scalding, searing: thermal dimension

Pinching, pressing, gnawing, cramping, crushing: dimensions of constrictive pressure

So already, right here in a suite of opening pages devoted to asserting otherwise, we see pain develop a language within language, or alongside it.

Early in *On Being Ill*, Virginia Woolf takes up a position that seems to seamlessly predict Scarry's self-contradictory one. Bemoaning the paucity of literature that explores pain or illness as its theme, in addition to failures of courage and imagination, Woolf points to what she calls the poverty of language itself. "Let a sufferer try to describe a pain in his head to a doctor and language at once runs dry. . . . He is forced to coin words himself, and, taking his pain in one hand, and a lump of pure sound in the other . . . so to crush them together that a brand new word in the end drops out."

In a kind of preemptive strike, she acknowledges our need to go straight to the well—to create new words—but the real action of the essay is to go ahead and do what everyone says can't be done. That is, through some alchemy of shifted perception and attention, to sweep the search-light of language across pain's murky terrain.

While Scarry attributes strange autonomies to pain—in just the first few pages of her introduction, pain *triumphs*, *achieves*, and *entails*—Woolf attributes strange autonomies to people in it. "How astonishing, when the lights of health go down," implies equally, how astonishing when the lights of ill-health come up, followed as it is by "the undiscovered countries that are disclosed . . . what wastes and deserts, what precipices and lawns sprinkled bright with flowers."

Pain and illness alter. They insist: "All day, all night the body intervenes." They invent: "blunts or sharpens, colors or discolors, turns to wax in the warmth of June, hardens to tallow in the murk of February." They isolate: "There is a virgin forest in each; a snowfield where even the print of birds' feet is unknown." They isolate: "Here we go alone, and like it better so." They invent: "other tastes assert themselves; sudden, fitful, intense." They insist: "This monster, the body, this miracle, its pain."

23

Exiled from the kingdom of health, the ill inherit a different land. What is shattered here, language or the perceived world language typically describes? Escapading through the slant studies of the pain- or illness-altered mind, transcribing its rapt, if mercurial, attentions to internal and external surrounds, it's as if Woolf stage-directs a play for which I've rehearsed all the parts:

That's me alone in the stranged room, feeling the action of eyeballs in eye sockets in the bone case of the face, watching light migrate across the wall.

Or, that leaf! That's my shadow leaf, so perfectly in place, so perfectly there, there, there. Now it's falling. Now absence perfect where it used to hang. ("This then has been going on all the time without our knowing it!")

Or, skimming as usual the usual devastating news, this day, this hour, this minute, that's me looking, really looking, at the faces and the prone bodies of people or animals or places in disarray on display, and before I know it, those are my dry sobs barking into thin air. ("This then has been going on . . .")

Soon, though, one leaves that "snowfield of the mind." Pain has turned its head (yours) in a different direction and so what that leaf that fell? Time to look away again from the news. Time again when "the hero becomes a white liquid with a sweet taste," for "with the hook of life still in us still we must wriggle." ("You have a quiet voice," the radio station's engineer remarks, adjusting my mike before an interview. "No," I say, "I just know when to keep it down.")

If, as Woolf seems to attest, pain is never just pain, but pain+, maybe migraine—that neurological disturbance cascading across the brain—is pain++. Disturbance disrupts: patterns, assumptions, habits, business as usual, normative modes of body and mind. Disrupted, realms are revealed: the revised realm created by what's newly added or absent, and the realm of revision—that is, the realm of knowing that the realm can be revised. For all of its undeniable impact and clatter, arguably migraine's most lasting effect is the revelation of this radical malleability: ours. *This, that, here, there, me, you*—all of it as if fashioned to a mechanism, a dial turning it up, a dial turning it down. You don't turn the dial, but the dial turns, and this ratcheting is you.

"The exquisite control (and, normally, latitude) of what we call 'health' may, paradoxically, be based on chaos," writes neurologist Oliver Sacks. "Perhaps this is especially true in patients with migraine. . . . Perhaps migraine itself, to use a favorite term of chaos theorists, can itself act as a 'strange attractor.'"

Nonpain Migraine Effects (mine):

Aural: acute sensitivity to sound, auditory hallucination (specific words, generalized murmur, hum, buzz, reverb and other effects), heightened sense of hearing

Cognitive: brain fog, decreased concentration, difficulty reading, diminished word retrieval, disorientation, dissociation, enhanced word retrieval, heightened reading acuity, increased concentration, temporal disruption

Digestive: appetite stimulation, appetite suppression, constipation, cravings, diarrhea, hypoglycemia, nausea, water retention, water shedding

Mood: accepting, agitated, antagonistic, apathetic, attuned, calm, cavalier, critical, curious, desperate, disinhibited, distant, energized, enervated, euphoric, generous, impatient, inhibited, irritable, loving, paranoid, passionate, risk-averse, risk-seeking, sad, sensitive, vacant, weepy

Olfactory: acute sensitivity to odors, heightened sense of smell, olfactory hallucination (pinewoods, dining hall, mother, toast, latrine)

Other: changes in blood pressure and circulation, increased perspiration, motion sickness, muscle soreness, muscle spasm, muscle weakness, thermal dysregulation

Tactile: altered sense of proprioception, choking sensation, feeling of mounting pressure in head (exacerbated by bending over, lying down, tipping chin up, or raising arms above head), heightened sense of touch, intolerance to anything touching neck or head, itchiness, skin sensitivity

Visual: acute sensitivity to light, altered color and light perception, blurred vision, hyperacuity of vision, visual hallucination (scintillations, shadows, pinpoints, flashes of light [usually blue])

24

Migraine says, Come on in, these doors are always open. Migraine says, Go ahead: count this, measure that while I flash around like schooling fish. Migraine says, If you come off the rails at 3:05 A.M. at an angle of thirty-three degrees and the dew point is dropping and the mockingbird just woke up, how long before you screech to a halt? Migraine says, Forget it, all forests *are* are trees. Migraine says, Is that your safe word or is that a new nickname for me? Migraine says, I'm the paint and, baby, you're the canvas. Migraine says, this cage is a mirror, this cage can make itself disappear; here, I will make a tray of you for the sky.

Waxing, waning, eclipsing—moon of your mornings, moon of your nights, migraine says, Now it's all black and white and gray, no more blue in here today. Migraine says, There was a symphony in here a minute ago, for a minute there all the colors of the rainbow were sitting on the knife's edge of this whole dull affair.

Now the storm goes away again in a series

of small, badly lit battle-scenes,

each in "Another part of the field."
(Elizabeth Bishop)

Prismatic is migraine's point of view. Through it, we see the world prismatically. In it, we see ourselves prismed. Does it sound like I want to have it all ways? It happens to happen all ways, sometimes in recognizable sequence, sometimes recombining endlessly according to who knows what. Migraine isn't receptacle; it's instrument, instant incubator throwing voices and light.

It was by accident that Donald Judd, famous for his sleek minimalist (he hated the term) sculptures exactingly displayed in dialogue with their environment, realized that a dimensional painting in the process of being hung belonged instead where it was, on the floor (unpredictable swerve). It was by design, however, that the foundation hosting me chose to locate its residency program in the tiny West Texas town where years earlier Judd headquartered himself after abandoning the New York art scene.

Seeking an alternative to typical galleries and museums for the display of his own and other artists' work, Judd built Chinati on the grounds of a former military base, beginning Marfa's (partial and ongoing) transformation from a little-known, former railroad, desert town to a renowned art outpost to which people travel from all over the world. I'm sure many factors informed the foundation's thinking: landscape, remoteness, size, sympathetic magic of various kinds. But there was also an intention for inter-play between artists and ideas, which is why, a few weeks into my time, I'm able to arrange for a series of private visits to Judd's *100 untitled works in mill aluminum*.

Housed in two former airplane hangars known as "the sheds" on the grounds of Chinati, *100 works* is a masterpiece of strict repetition as a means to infinite variation, of art whose medium is perception, of context and frame, of light. "Each of the 100 works has the same outer dimensions (41 × 51 × 72 inches), although the interior is unique in every piece." If migraine's prism could be painless, if migraine mind could be prismed through the lens of a hundred brushed aluminum boxes reflecting desert earth and sky, it would look like this.

Welcome to the amplified inner chamber, entering seems to speak. Your breath is a bellows. Here in the silence, sound when it rings out rings through the full field of its rising and falling to the vibrating ends you can feel but no longer hear. Light is captured, now it holds you hostage, makes sparkle, makes strange, slams darkly bright. Sometimes what you see is a ramp, sometimes a precipice, sometimes a hollow, sometimes a screen, a scrim, a veil, a mirror. Sometimes what is present goes absent and what you see disguises itself as nothing at all. Out there, beyond—the hovel huts we eat and drink and die in, the cars speeding by and the birds that dive—who cares, let them, we are here now and everywhere else is elsewhere. Hallowed hall of the inside call: we could stand here staring all day, and sometimes we do.

Or, welcome to the play. The set is these objects on this stage. The stage is this place you find yourself standing, and also your mind. Today's performance, like every day's performance, stars your perception unfolding in the loop that is your body feeding your mind feeding your body feeding your mind. In space. In time.

25

Private temple where I go to find god or no god, self or no self, I'd rather not share the boxes with anyone and, miraculously, I don't have to, solitary worship a gift of the residency I'm on, the leave I've taken. At the beginning of each new semester, though, I make a ritual of taking my students to *The Color Inside*, a James Turrell Skyspace installed on the roof of the University of Texas's Student Activities Building.

The Skyspace is a naked-eye observatory in the heart of the main campus, where visitors view the sky through an opening in the ceiling called an oculus. During sunrise and sunset, colored lights illuminate the walls and contrast the natural skylight in the oculus. This affects the way we see the sky and produces the experience of James Turrell's art. While Turrell considers

his art only visible during sunrise and sunset,
the Skyspace is available for observation dur-
ing the day.

We go at sunset, watch for an hour and eleven
minutes as an orchestrated sequence of colored lights rewrites the way our eyes read the
color of the actual sky. Turrell has done his
research: optics, color theory, physics of light,
physiology of perception—brain and eye. Cast
upward from hidden holds, projected color
creeps across, quickly saturates the pristine
white walls and ceiling framing the oculus.
It starts slowly, it's under way before we fully
know, and then it's in full swing. Our carved
portion of oval sky has shifted register, degree:
ordinary blue (beautiful enough) grows deeper,
electric, morphs turquoise, celadon, emerald,
aqua, cerulean, celery; fades dove gray, then
white, stone, maybe, beige, pumpkin, mud
brown, now black, now back: blue again, our
feet touch ground, then off, onward, elsewhere,
gone. Sometimes—chance operation—a flock
of birds or an airplane floats by.

Framing the experience through a question—
How do we make something out of nothing?—foregrounding the processes of perception and
their malleability, my notes read not unlike a
discussion of migraine: All we do is perceive.
Everything is relative. One thing (re)invents
the next. We are always translating. Perception
is a form of translation. Language is a form of
translation. Everything associates. The brain is
a simile-making machine. Everything exists in
time. Everything creates its own time line.

"My work is more about your seeing than it is
about my seeing," Turrell explains, showing us
the pliancy of the mechanics by which we navigate and name, by which we make and are made.
A romp. "This affects the way we see the sky . . ."

I tell them it's funny: He turns the blue sky
brown! Didn't the surprise geese crack you up?
Notice how long he withholds red, then really lets
us have it. I tell them it's political: he's showing
us exactly how much to believe our own eyes. I
tell them it's personal: we compare notes—when
the sky pushed in, when it pulled out, when the
walls fell away, how our vision spun, if yellow has

a secret or a scent, whether the oculus is a pupil, a periscope, a microscope, a bird's egg, a god's eye—and discover how idiosyncratically each of our bodies and minds "produces the experience."

26

In *Strange Tools: Art and Human Nature*, philosopher Alva Noë posits that underlying the innate human urge to make and experience art is not the pursuit of an object (noun), but the engagement of a process (verb). Specifically, that art-making is a form of research.

Most artists would agree, I think: the product may be what's prayed for, but the process is what's lived. What strikes me as novel in Noë's approach is to frame art-making and the urgency that instigates it specifically as an essential kind of research, a vital practice of investigation into ourselves and the world. "Art provides us an opportunity to catch ourselves in the act of achieving our conscious lives, of bringing the world into focus for perceptual (and other forms of) consciousness," Noë writes, in response to which I think: likewise. That is, migraine may be unwelcome and it may not mean, but it is a means of research into the range of us.

"The law is on the side of the normal," says Virginia Woolf, and who would argue? In pain or ill, "we cease to be soldiers in the army of the upright; we become deserters." But desertion by means of conscription insists we join up as much as we leave behind. Unsurprisingly, perhaps, our novel rations comprise not only our altered perception but our altered relationship to language, too. "In illness words seem to possess a mystic quality . . . with the police off duty, we creep beneath . . . and the words give up their scent and distill their flavor."

Intralanguage, extralanguage, words that give up their scent. Poetry is a genre "in which the rules of language and narrative can be subverted," *The New York Times* helpfully explains on the occasion of basketball star Kobe Bryant's retirement announcement via poem. "Poetry is the place where language gets to be as strange as it actually is," says Mary. Poems are things made of language striving to uncover, engage, even reinvent the way language works and thereby the way it works on us—to reveal and flourish via malleability: language's, ours.

In the conversation of contemporary American poetry, no word is more frequently used or less conclusively defined than *lyric*, which is sometimes an adjective, sometimes a noun. Attributed multiple and often contradictory meanings over the centuries, these days, it speaks variously to immediacy, intensity, intimacy, subjectivity, and the expression of revelatory thought or feeling in burstlike or fragmented form. Sometimes it's understood as the voice of the poet talking to herself under the normal conditions of an individual's private, fractured thoughts; sometimes as the personal expression of a fictional speaker; sometimes as the performance of the mind in solitary speech. Or some combination thereof. Coherence and cohesiveness can be characteristic, but so, too, dissociation and fragmentation. We say lyric leap, lyric voice. Do we say lyric mind?

"Sappho is simultaneously losing composure and composing herself, falling apart in the poem and coming together as a poem that seems to speak, with heightened eloquence," writes Longinus in the seventeenth century of the Archaic Greek poet widely considered to be the wellspring of the Western lyric tradition. "From this accidental peculiarity of ancient writers, the criticks deduce the rules of lyrick poetry, which they have set free from all the laws by which other compositions are confined, and allow to neglect the niceties of transition, to start into remote digressions, and to wander without restraint from one scene of imagery to another," writes Rambler in the eighteenth century. In the late twentieth century, Richard Fineman proposes "a new model of lyric subjectivity in which the divided subject of modernity 'experiences himself as his difference from himself.'" Sound familiar?

27

"Was it cathartic to write that?" a well-intentioned audience member asks after I read an excerpt from an early draft.

> *Catharsis (n): from the Greek to cleanse, to purge*
>
> a. *Purgation of the excrements of the body; esp. evacuation of the bowels*
>
> b. *Purification of the emotions by vicarious experience, esp. through drama*
>
> c. *The process of relieving an abnormal excitement by reestablishing the association of the emotions with the memory or idea of the event which was the first cause of it, and of eliminating it by abreaction*

Later, Dot and I discuss whether the question is a gendered one—would a man be asked the same? Consider: women and the body, women and emotions, the so-called Confessional poets, women and their creative hobbies, isn't that nice. Consider: female equals emotion; male equals intellect. See also: hysteria and other "female pathologies." And: conditions once attributed to "maternal failure," including anorexia, autism, homosexuality, schizophrenia, and sexual deviance. Consider, too:

One in four women has had a migraine. (NPR)

For every man with a migraine, three women are struck. (UCLA Newsroom)

Of the more than 36 million Americans afflicted with migraine, 27 million are women. (Migraine Research Foundation)

Why? Historically far worse, the range—and, in some cases, the content—of reasons still bandied about are sometimes maddening. Let's go with this one, relatively neutral and seemingly grounded in our best current understanding:

*Dr. Andrew Charles directs the Head-
ache Research and Treatment Program in
the UCLA Department of Neurology. He
describes what occurs during a migraine as a
"spectacular neuro-physiological event" that
involves bursts of electrical activity that start
in the vision center of the brain. . . . The brain
activity then travels like a wave across the landscape of the brain. What triggers a migraine
is nearly as complicated as the migraine itself.
There are environmental changes like sounds,
light, smells and movement. There are genes;
migraine risk is hereditary. But there is one
major trigger, and this is why women have so
many more migraines than men. Neurologist
Jan Lewis Brandes, founder of the Nashville
Neuroscience Group, says migraines can be
triggered by hormonal fluctuation.* (NPR)

(But we knew that.)

"Ask me in six months to a year," I answer,
trying to be generous while I deflect. "No,"
I might more honestly have said. Or, "I don't
understand the question."

Denial and compartmentalization have long been my primary means of coping, and as far as I can tell, they've mostly served me well. That is, they have delivered me reasonably close to my desired ends: a life that accommodates as necessary but does not orient itself around migraine. In other words, a life.

I've written on migraine as on a drug. I've written through migraine as through fog or storm. I've written with migraine as with a jagged star stuck in my eye. Sometimes I've knowingly imported the sensibilities of migraine mind into the poems I write. Other times, I assume, I've done so unknowingly. In any given moment, my relationship to language may be actively metabolizing migraine, and when migraine isn't currently present, that relationship is still shaped, like anyone's, by my accumulated experience—its form as much as its content. I gave a version of my affliction to a character once, a displaced traveler studying moths, obsessed with seeing and stricken by pain, dissembling in the process. Some readers have praised what they see as the book's foray into science fiction, and I'm not ungrateful, but no, this strangeness is ours—it comes from inside, not from out there.

The brain has corridors—surpassing

Material Place—

Ourself behind ourself, concealed—

Should startle most— (Emily Dickinson)

Mostly, though, uninterested in personal revelation, unwilling to yield even more precious time and attention, and inchoately flustered or dismayed by nearly everything I read on the subject, I've avoided it. For years, my policy was a kind of zero tolerance vigilantly pursued: Give the monster nothing, not one minute more than what by stealth or by force it took. Accommodate what must be accommodated, but volunteer for nothing: not deep research, not support group esprit de corps, not even, really, a moment's reflection. Another form of magical thinking, a felt superstition: don't let the gods mistake your intent. So why am I writing this?

28

Through the stock footage of memory unnamed three-legged dogs hop-run across snapshot terrains—no one dog in particular, a montage, almost, a kind of highlight reel. This spring's midsize terrier romping along a rocky trail bordering Inks Lake. Last summer's black Lab skipping across an emerald lawn in the Berkshires. Summer before, a carefully coiffed goldendoodle foreleg-rowing down Commercial Street, withered hind legs pinned to a skateboardlike contraption.

Further back, the motley ones making it somehow sprightly in the feral pack of abandoned pets and their ragged offspring garbage-picking at the dump on Paros. Others, the unplaced ones of childhood, vividly or only barely recalled, but regularly during the long hours of the treatment years spent IV-ing in dimly lit rooms with other intractably afflicted people whom I wanted to end up nothing like. One of the sick, I found in the sick no viable model. Or, more gently put, that snowfield was one I had to go alone.

If my instinct was animal—as soon as pain lifted, I fled its barbed pen; as soon as it lowered, I paced its razor-wire perimeter or hunkered down along its edge—my aesthetic was, too, and so these memory dogs, never consciously chosen but repeatedly conjured, became my model. At the time, I thought it was for the stalwart way they adjusted to reality's impositions but otherwise went about the merry business of their lives. In retrospect, I realize that one of the primary features distinguishing my beloved three-leggeds from the suffering people I found myself among was the fact that with words, at least, dogs can't speak.

"God must love you very much" is what Colin said the nun told him, age seven or eight, when he fell and split his chin walking up the marble steps to receive First Communion, blood everywhere. (Pain as evidence.) We were in the blackened shell of his family home a few weeks after his schizophrenic brother had burned it down for the second time, a few weeks before the contractors would rebuild it again. Sixteen at the time, both of us lying to our parents about where we were, this was the germinal ground of our ill-fated love affair, for me a bitterly self-destructive relationship my mother later blamed for the origin of my migraines. (Pain as proof.)

"Do you pray?" he asked accusingly. "Sort of," I answered. "What for?" he demanded. I was fortunate: healthy, mostly happy, well loved by family and friends, but not by him, which, I think, is why I was there. "Please protect and preserve me and those that I love," I mumbled, chagrined to be saying aloud what was only ever a silent incantation. "Must be nice," he said, voice dripping with disdain (another way grief goes awry), which I understood as intended: Isn't it pretty to think so?

Affliction as mark, suffering as love, love as suffering inflicted or affliction withstood. "Not I," said the duck and all the other barnyard animals whom the hen asked for help in the children's story. "No thank you," wailed the toddler once upon a feverish time as I approached with a rectal thermometer. What if we don't like the options we're given? "No thank you," he screamed.

What if I don't like the options I'm given? Rather, what if no viable options are given? Neither refusal (impossible) nor embrace (unthinkable). According to Boolean logic, in which the values of given variables are true or false, Logical Nor is "a logical operation on two logical values, typically the values of two propositions, that produces a value of true if and only if both operands are false." Sometimes this action is called "joint denial."

29

"Every rule admits exceptions," cautions John M. Lee in "Some Remarks on Writing Mathematical Proofs," a style guide I find eerily apt just now. "Although you might initially construct your proof as a sequence of terse symbolic statements, when you write it up you should use complete sentences organized into paragraphs," because, he reminds us, "your goal is to communicate to a human reader." Further advice includes:

> *Don't be stingy with intuitive explanations of what's going on and why. . . . Include motivation. . . . Use the first person singular sparingly, but if you're really referring only to yourself, it's better to go ahead and use "I" so you don't sound like the Queen of England.*

> *Ask yourself What does it mean? Why is it*
> *true? Include more than just the logic.*

Similarly, in "Ten Tips for Writing Mathematical Proofs," Katharine Otts suggests, "If you get stuck, it is often helpful to turn to definitions." And, "Do not use symbols when you write your proof. This is ambiguous and your reader will not be sure what it means."

Catching up after both of us having been through a difficult time, I propose to Matthea an idea for a graphic novel–style reference book entitled *An Incomplete Field Guide to Accompanying the Visibly and Invisibly Wounded.* One per page, each entry would briefly describe a situation and offer related advice on interacting with loved ones, or even acquaintances, in pain (depression, grief, trauma, illness, injury). Gleaned from the data—our own and others'—of having done and been done unto, we brainstorm something succinct, with illustrations.

Example: If your loved one is suffering an acute bout within the context of chronic depression, don't choose the moment after he tells you he can't get out of bed and he's afraid this may be the one that never lifts to grab your sneakers and head to the gym.

Example: If your loved one suffers from migraines that sometimes make her irritable, don't ask, "Do you have a headache?" whenever she gets angry about anything.

Example: If your loved one is grieving a loss due to suicide, don't joke about jumping off a building.

Example: When your loved one says she feels alone, do stay in the room.

Example: If crippling fatigue is a symptom of your friend's condition, don't tell him you keep staying up late or that you've really been pushing it at hot yoga lately or you only got seven hours when you're used to eight, so you know just how he feels, join the club, really, you're just exhausted.

Example: If an author's work reveals that she lives with a painful condition, don't feel compelled to approach her after the reading to say how glad you are that you don't suffer this particular affliction—the author is glad for you, too.

30

"Organisms exist within systems of organization—it's the condition of ourselves—art disrupts these," Alva Noë remarks during a talk on the heels of visiting *100 works*, where I've been stealing ecstatic time. Hosted by the local bookstore, where I happened to be browsing, the conversation between Noë and author Lawrence Weschler is bookended by poems: "A Jar in Tennessee" (Stevens) and "Guard Duty" (Tranströmer). "Art/migraine disrupts habitual choreographies, it reorganizes us, it reorganizes time," read my scribbled notes. I've lost track of which words are theirs, which mine. "I am the turnstile," the Tranströmer poem ends.

Donald Judd's boxes bring into high relief, they lay bare point of view, temporality, associative function, aesthetic pleasure, control and chance, shadow and light, source and reflection, the changeability inherent to each. Making physically manifest before and within us the mechanisms of perception, the exquisite illusions of apprehension, the shifting kaleidoscope that is any moment of our knowing, their reflection-refraction-illusion assertions form a knife's edge, a vision ledge, an alternate take and another and another—the multiplicity of any knowable thing.

Forgive me, ghost of Donald Judd and your earthly keepers of the flame, but so, too, pain, so, too, migraine. I don't mean to reduce your masterpiece of specificity, of ecstatic geometry, to the confines of an agenda, mine. I mean the opposite. I mean that by articulating, distilling, amplifying, revealing the glory process of perception, the boxes speak to everything—certainly not only to pain, maybe not even to pain in particular, but to pain, too.

Scratch that. Every bridge feels insufficient. What I mean is that like the sheds, migraine is a space you enter and are enveloped by and it is a different version of the world in there, where perception itself is an identifiable orchestration in full swing, and all the familiar and all the strange, the invented and the reflected and the revealed take up their parts and, like music, unfold in time, but a form of time contained by the architecture of certain stabilities so you can not quite rewind or repeat but continue playing or step back into the playing, which is always playing until you step back out of it and in some ways it stops and in other ways it keeps going.

When I was nine or ten years old, I had a habit of hiding in the den before supper. Lying on the couch without turning on the lights as evening fell, I would hold perfectly still thinking over and over in my mind, *Things will never be exactly the same ever again*. The clang of pots in the kitchen, the any-minute-now call to gather around the bright table, to leave behind the moment held in stillness—even though I'd done it yesterday and would do it again tomorrow, nothing would ever be the same.

I took up this practice around the time I was trying to understand the concept of infinity. The best I could do was to think *And on and on and on* for as long as I could stand to and then, having become distracted or bored, whenever I remembered to pick up the dropped refrain, to imagine that the whole space between—the space of my forgetting—had been filled with it, too, *And on and on* going forward, endlessly. But back to the couch. All this time I've thought I was thinking about time, about loss inherent to time, rehearsing nostalgia, maybe. Now I think, yes, but also: this was the beginning of my research.

Exquisite mirrors, miraculous translators, more than anything, Judd's boxes are perception-revelation machines. They provide a neutral field where the mind manifests—delicately dropping its veils, revealing its gears, their actions. "Stop anthropomorphizing the glacier," I tell Dahr after reading the introduction he's drafted for the book about climate disruption he's spending his residency time working on. "The glacier didn't invite or disinvite you, it doesn't want or not want you, it didn't decide to spare or to take you in the first place. The glacier doesn't know you. The glacier doesn't care. The glacier is a phenomenon." In this way, the glacier is like pain and pain is like the boxes. The beauty, the love, is in what we perceive.

31

Across the street, Mary's writing through, writing to, a different kind of pain. We don't talk about it, but catty-corner in our little houses, sketching words on cloud-white pages, or walking side by side in the burnt-gold desert, we help each other by virtue of juxtaposition.

I'm circling the pain of presence; she's circling the pain of absence. As if peering through one-way mirrors, we access the altered aperture of a different kind of grief. That is, in each other, we make out a version of pain we're not presently suffering, and this is good to remember, a kind of grace through negative space, like that provided by the aggressive tom turkey we've seen patrolling the neighborhood but by whom we've so far been spared: here is a pain I am not right now suffering, a pain that has not come to pass.

In this slant way, I think, I return to her the body of the moment and she returns to me the body freed from it. This doesn't change the pain we're in, but it changes something. At least, one way or another, I'm brought around to a different feeling of duration: *Darling, even knowing, of course I would have had you.*

Juxtaposition, collision, accidental swerve. Consciousness as perception, perception as apprehension of unlike. Exile from the known as conscription into other knowing. All of these refractions describe a necessary devotion to the generative power of creative friction—creative as in creator, friction as in pain. We experience the new as pain and pain ushers us into the new. But how long does the new remain revelatory once revealed? How long do we get to hold its novel gift of body in body, of mind in mind?

"Once mastered, learning of all kinds becomes unconscious and automatic," writes Siri Hustvedt in a recent essay on gendered literature and the feminization of feeling. "Consciousness, it seems, is parsimonious, reserved for dealing not with routine and predictable perceptions in our

lives, but with what is novel and unpredictable."
According to contemporary neuroscience, this
process is called "pruning." Especially in infant
and early childhood development, but recently
and radically reassessed as a lifelong practice,
in the forest of the brain neural branches are
established and reinforced through experience,
while unused boughs fall away.

It's a process that saves us, on which we rely: so
densely thicketed is the brain we are born with,
so cacophonous the woods within and around
us, we can't see through the trees; we can't even
see the trees. Arguably, in this way, we arrive
uniquely helpless as mammals go: underde-
veloped and overexposed. (A newborn fawn is
capable of running at nearly full speed within
minutes of its birth, etc.) But also, arguably, in
this way we are uniquely adapted by virtue of
being adaptable. Scientists now posit this neural
prematurity not as an unfortunate price to pay
for the unforgiving geometry of uprightness—
hip width to skull diameter—but as a wily evolutionary advantage.

"The brain is literally molded by experience: every sight, sound, and thought leaves an imprint on specific neural circuits, modifying the way future sights, sounds, and thoughts will be registered," writes Lise Eliot, a neuroscientist whose research focuses on learning. "Brain hardware is not fixed, but living, dynamic tissue that is constantly updating itself to meet the sensory, motor, emotional, and intellectual demands at hand." In the version of our story that she tells, we enter the arena helpless by design: still meaningfully malleable and ready to be wired up advantageously in concert with our particular environment. By arriving and to some extent remaining unbuilt, we are built for perception, for experience. But this gain is made of loss: unused branches fall away.

32

Like most good metaphors, pruning works on multiple levels, marrying the primal forest of our ancestral imagination to the living woods around us, and to the newest visions available to us via the prophecies of instruments. Seen through high-powered microscopes, individual neurons look like trees, leafless and many-boughed; groups of them look like forests.

"There's no distinction between painting a landscape of a forest and a landscape of the brain," notes Greg Dunn, former neuroscientist turned artist specializing in renderings of brain and spinal cord cells. In his new work, as in his old, Dunn is aware of the need to resist the gravitational pull of the rote habits of mind Siri Hustvedt cautions against. Apparently, it's difficult to reproduce accurately the randomness inherent to the way neurons branch, so Dunn has developed a technique of blowing ink onto paper to compensate for the mind's bias toward pattern. "If you try to paint neurons by hand," he says, "you adhere to all kinds of unconscious rules."

In any case, it's how we're built. At the most basic level, failure to prune—to select and sort, to predict based on past experience—results in an incapacity to perceive properly due to an excess of perception, something like a neurological traffic jam, which is how sensory processing disorder is described by A. Jean Ayres, one of its pioneering researchers. Likewise, failure to prune at the level of basic cognition—to select and sort, to predict based on past experience—results in an overwhelmed and misfiring mind, one unable to cope with its surroundings and incapable of making decisions.

If we're to be open to the truly novel, we can't continually be accosted by the ever-repeating new of standard-fare sensory input. Perception and consciousness must be organized into predictable patterns and reasonable expectations (fathomable portions): we must be able to fill in the blank. Faced every minute with a million *ands*, *alsos*, and *elsewheres*, we have to know in any given instant where our attention is and is not really required. On the one hand, this describes a kind of passivity, a type of forgetting, a way of unseeing. On the other hand, this describes a type of activity, a kind of making, a means of envisioning.

"Perception is by its very nature conservative and biased, a form of typecasting that helps us make sense of the world," Hustvedt concludes, simultaneously echoing scientific findings and tracing *clinamen*'s evolving definition from accident-based creation to bias-twisted conclusion. "We do not passively receive information from the world but are rather creative interpreters of it." Science writer and onetime lab technician Jonah Lehrer describes it as the brain "refining a set of cellular forecasts," a framework that seems to encompass the possibilities held in each hand. To predict the weather is a narrowing down, a reliance on past experience and available data. But it is also expansive, an act of imagination. And, though irresistible and sometimes important, it's frequently revealed as an act of folly.

So reliant is the brain upon the anticipated patterns and predictions of its forecasting, when an expectation goes unmet, it sends out a neurochemical flare called a "prediction-error signal." At the start of each semester, in a thinly veiled attempt to undermine clichéd habits of mind and beseech openness in response to art, paraphrasing Lehrer, I offer up my understanding of the phenomenon.

For the sake of efficiency, I say, the human brain works in repeated patterns and pathways. It can't pay attention to everything all at once, so it relies on these pattern-based expectations and repetitions, which, once established and subsequently provoked, allow the brain to simply fill in the rest without having to really notice everything every time. When the brain encounters a break in pattern, an unmet expectation, it reacts with a prediction-error signal, a kind of chemical gong struck. We can't control the fact that we have this reflex, but we can control our response to it. (Note the hopeful conclusion.)

Lehrer himself talks about dopamine in lab monkeys rewarded with apple juice:

> *Once this simple pattern was learned, the monkey's dopamine neurons became exquisitely sensitive to variations on it. If the cellular predictions proved correct, and the reward arrived right on time, then the primate experienced a brief surge of dopamine, the pleasure of being right. However, if the pattern was violated—if the tone was played but the juice never arrived—then the monkey's dopamine neurons decreased their firing rate. This is known as the prediction-error signal. The monkey felt upset because its predictions of juice were wrong.*

In truth, I included the last line above almost entirely for aesthetic reasons, but it possesses relevant pathos, too, illustrative as it is of the poor pattern-seeking reader bereft of juice every time a poem does something truly unexpected. Bereft or, possibly, ecstatic? I don't know if it's accurate, but I always claim that while we can't choose whether or not to have the neurological response, the fact of its existence doesn't dictate the quality of its experience. Aren't we all familiar with a range of responses to the new, the unexpected, both in ourselves and in one another? Fear and loathing sometimes, but sometimes joy and exaltation, too. Either way, we're paying attention. "The brain is designed to amplify the shock of these mistaken predictions," Lehrer writes. "Whenever it experiences something unexpected the cortex immediately takes notice."

Hustvedt turns to primates, too. "Rote activities call for minimal consciousness, but if while standing in my kitchen, I turn and see a gorilla pounding on the window, full awareness is imperative. More often than not, when gorillas are not pounding on our kitchen windows, we see what we expect to see." But what if the brain itself is the source of the unexpected? What if migraine is the gorilla pounding at the glass, breaking patterns, breaching expectations? What if regularly the gorilla comes to call?

33

"Other than that, Mrs. Lincoln, how did you like the play?" is an expression my mother is fond of and one with which she not infrequently wraps up our conversations about my migraine-stricken day or week or month when I've signaled that I want to get off the phone. Here, denial is a pivot. *Other than that*, acknowledges *that* in the same instant it shifts away from it. Interestingly, Mrs. Lincoln isn't the one in denial—at least not yet—her interlocutor is, proffering an invitation to the aggrieved to enter an attentive space of after or elsewhere.

"It's the hoariest sick joke in America," claims Timothy Noah in a recent article subtitled "Was the Play that Ended Lincoln's Life Any Good?" "By now, it isn't even a joke; it's become a familiar way to complain that undue attention is being given to some frivolous aspect of an otherwise grim and urgent matter," he continues, and from there, with no apparent irony, goes on to do just that, asking, "What sort of aesthetic experience occupied the Great Emancipator's final hours?" A preposterous question, to be sure. Also a ruefully loving one? One in the spirit of which we not infrequently get on with our days?

"Both/and," my therapist likes to say when we're talking, as we often do, about living with pain. "It's true," she confirms, when I ask if the therapeutic understanding of denial is still overwhelmingly negative. "Denial is considered a defense, a lower-order one at that." (What constitutes a higher-order defense? Humor.) The spin is, she explains, that defenses, though sometimes necessary, are maladaptive, unhealthy: they're something we use until we can face reality. "Denial assumes the psyche can't handle it, whatever *it* is."

After years of letting me refer to my strategy for coping with the ongoingness of the migraines as if it's an established concept, she admits that I've invented my own term, or at least my own usage: "functional denial," a kind of selective refusal to integrate. This strategy accounts for my real beef with counting and accounting, case histories and forward projections—they disrupt my invented weather of plausible deniability, of gentle, amnesiac leanings cultivated as coping mechanism but also maybe a by-product of the present-tense-on-repeat iterations of the migraines themselves, which come, go, cascade of what only ever appears to be their own accord. Today? Yes, today.

"The closest concept we have to what you do is called 'adaptive denial,'" she tells me when I ask, some twelve years into our conversation. "Adaptive denial says, 'Okay, this is a tool I'm going to choose to use to help me contain something or manage it.' I decided pretty early on with you to just leave it alone because it seemed to be working. Anyway," she continues, "things are rapidly changing. Our concept of denial comes out of the late nineteenth and early twentieth centuries and is considered psychological, neurotic, not neurophysical which is where the most exciting work is being done these days."

Demerol, depression. Delirium, depersonalization. Demons, dentistry. Book after book in my micro migraine library skips over denial completely. But I find plenty of mention of it elsewhere.

"Denial is an ego defense mechanism that operates unconsciously to resolve emotional conflicts, and to allay anxiety by refusing to perceive the more unpleasant aspects of external reality," writes clinical psychologist Kathy McMahon, regarding attitudes toward climate change in "Exploring Emotional Reactions to Peak Oil." In keeping with standard interpretations, McMahon characterizes denial as an agent of inertia, even paralysis. Refusing to take in the unpleasant reality not only obviates the need for action; it makes action impossible: we can't act to solve what we convincingly deny.

According to this logic, a breaking down of denial is a necessary step toward action, but what if such a breaking down leads instead to breakdown? What if sometimes it is denial's gloss, its preservation of "a sense of order and security and also a sense of innocence," that makes a refusal of paralysis possible? "It serves to soften the blow of such a startling and unfathomable truth," even McMahon concedes. And: "there exists within us a complicated emotional storm."

34

"Our first problem arises from the word *migraine*," Oliver Sacks proclaims at the outset of *Migraine*, but this is the least of my problems with a book I've picked up and angrily tossed aside more than a dozen times. Originally published in 1970, the idiosyncratic study combining patient histories, historical and contemporary research findings, and interpretative, often highly subjective analysis was the first of many books by the neurologist turned author, who was later dubbed "the poet laureate of contemporary medicine" by *The New York Times*.

"A migraine is a physical event which may also be from the start, or later become, an emotional or symbolic event," Sacks writes in his "Historical Introduction," marking migraine as "the prototype of a psycho-physiological reaction."

Despite the almost fifty years and nearly unfathomable advances in technology and medicine
separating this utterance from my reading now
(yet another attempt to due-diligence my way
through), I can't forgive him or his Freudian
henchmen for imagining, for example, *aggressive migraine*, in which unmet emotional needs
are sublimated into migraines deployed as
"implicit assaults or vengeful attacks," or *emu-
lative migraine*, in which a child manifests "an
ambivalent and malignant identification with a
migrainous parent; joining the parent in illness,
competing with him, hoisting him with his own
migrainous petard."

But beneath the damning presumptions and
exasperating insults embedded in its elaborate
administration, Sacks's study serves as a kind
of collective trial record shot through with the
glimmering testimony of myriad unmade mys-
tics, patient-witnesses, migraineurs condemned
to carry out sentences of embodied devotions
they did not choose through the procedural
courts of their days. Exuberant researcher, fellow
(albeit exceptional) sufferer, well-intentioned if
sometimes catastrophic almost-friend, Sacks's

voice and its cacophony of inheritance nearly drown out the truth-telling chorus, but theirs is the real record we're left holding in the end—literally.

Freed from the regular-rain trajectories of rote categorizations and biased interpretations, it is the study's inherently fragmented end matter that sings: indexes and appendixes, glossaries of terms and case histories, testimonies pulled from the historical record, even reproduced drawings depicting the migrainous visions of the twelfth-century French nun Hildegard of Bingen, originally rendered by her own hand.

In Figure IIA, the background is formed of shimmering stars set upon wavering concentric lines.

In Figure IIB, a shower of brilliant stars (phosphenes) is extinguished after its passage.

In Figures IIC and IID, Hildegard depicts typically migrainous fortification figures radiating from a central point, which, in the original, is brilliantly luminous and coloured.

Amid countless historical descriptions of visions, the origins of which are impossible to ascertain ("whether the experience represents a hysterical or psychotic ecstasy, the effects of intoxication, or an epileptic or migrainous manifestation"), Sacks and others before him declare Hildegard a bona fide lifelong migraineur whose visions were aura-induced.

> *I saw a great star most splendid and beautiful, and with it an exceeding multitude of falling stars . . . And suddenly they were all annihilated, being turned into black coals.*

> *The light which I see is not located, but yet is more brilliant than the sun, nor can I examine its height, length or breadth, and I name it "the cloud of living light."*

> *The visions which I saw I beheld neither in sleep, nor in dreams, nor in madness, nor with my carnal eyes, nor with the ears of the flesh, nor in hidden places; but wakeful, alert, and with the eyes of the spirit and the inward ears, I perceived them in open view and according to the will of God.*

From Sacks's language stripped of context, its routinized patterns, I fashion my own ancilla, assembling my own familiar-strange, sometimes numinous lists:

> Aura: *consciousness doubled in, daymares in, delirium in, dreamy state in, forced reminiscence in, giggling in, hallucinations in, horror in, music in, nightmare and, paintings of, trance*

> Aura: *bagel vision, cinematographic vision, Lilliputian vision, mosaic vision, zoom vision*

> Migraine: *abdominal, annual, arousal, brief maniacal, circumstantial, classical, cluster, common, common and classical, looming, red, regressive, sudden, Sunday or Sabbatical, white*

> Migraine: *as of ants on the skin, forced thinking, hatred of light, hatred of sound, an odd dancing, a sort of twinkling, a special vocabulary, strange smells, we speak of phantoms*

> And other indexes: *acquired, airy, anger and, Aristotle, barbiturates, borderlands of, catharsis, chaotic state of, chemical theories*

*of, constellations, déjà vu, delirium, elec-
trical theories of, figments, filigrees, flicker,
gender as factor in, history, holocrania, hun-
ger, hysteria, inheritance, jamais vu, Joan of
Arc, light: flickering, music: hallucinations
of, music: provokes, music: soothes, nerve
storms, noise, nonlinear dynamics, perceptual units, predisposition, pregnancy and,
recent advances, self as, spectra: pericentral
and rainbow, survival value, symbolic meaning, sympathetic theory of, ur-, weather and,
wonder*

35

The counting of days, the accounting of hours, is necessarily a mortal finitude. Looking back may have its hazards, but peering into the future does, too. This is the treacherous dovetail: denial may be how I've managed migraine, but migraine is what undoes my denial. In those dimly lit treatment rooms and outside of them, I learned there's no good time to be stricken and no preparation for being struck. Vulnerability jars into every cell, into every sense of past and future self: I know my weakness, I taste regularly the salt of overwhelming pain on my tongue, and through the present of this pain—*the*, *my*—I slide into the possibility of others—*your*, *his*, *our*.

Prediction, prognosis, prophecy: the forward projection may be something we lean toward, even yearn for, but fortune-telling flirtations aside, concrete prognostications are something we tend to avoid, even in the protected realms of our imaginations. In other words, distressing as it may be to crunch the numbers of stricken hours past, it's something else entirely to calculate those to come.

"We've been coming here for forty years," says my mother, inhaling deeply of salt and scrub pine, ocean to the left, lighthouse to the right. We're standing on a small promontory, fenced in and adorned with a plaque explaining how fifteen years earlier they moved the lighthouse fifty yards back from the eroding dune's edge. How long before they'll need to move it again?

Since the dawn of his relational consciousness, I've worried toward the moment when the development of my son's analytic mind would require an introduction to certain facts (tragic knowing): about me, about the world into which he'd been ushered. "The good thing is that even though they cause me a lot of pain, the headaches don't actually hurt me," I find myself saying periodically, aware that I'm making little sense. "I mean, they don't harm me," I attempt to clarify. "They won't kill me; they'll never be what makes me die."

"Pain is always different to the sufferer," writes Alphonse Daudet in *In the Land of Pain*, his unfinished autobiographical novel, "but loses its originality for those around him. Everyone will get used to it except me."

"I have a headache," he says when it's time to do his homework. "Water, get me water," he moans, flinging himself across the bed, "and migraine meds!" Then he pops up, smiling. "Mama, what I think of migraine is like a flock of migrating birds coming and hitting your head—not on the outside, but on the inside of your mind."

36

"Would you give up a freedom in exchange for a constraint if it meant you could be free of grief?" a bereaved ornithologist asks mid-soliloquy in the third act of *Now Now Oh Now*, a new play by the ensemble-based theater collective Rude Mechs. Mostly, she's been talking about beauty, how we respond to it, and arguing for Darwin's lesser-known theory of aesthetic selection.

Later I learn she's riffing on a theory developed by evolutionary biologist Richard Prum, professor of Ornithology and head curator of Vertebrate Zoology at Yale's Peabody Museum of Natural History. Workshopping a different play during a residency at the university, members of the theater company crossed paths with Prum when he stopped by to say he'd enjoyed their performance and, in conversation, shared something of his own work. His reimagining of questions such as how and why a finch might select for yellow struck a chord with one of the playwrights, becoming the seed of a new play, the one I was watching.

Survival of the fittest as macho competition plays out violently across our culture in its very architecture and self-image, its sense even of what's right, but, the grieving scientist reminds us, there's something dangerously occluded, something fundamentally incomplete about our definition of fitness. Often it's chance that leads to survival, and frequently it's beauty that draws us, that constitutes the so-called fitness to which we respond, for which we select—for instance, color; for instance, song.

Would you give up a freedom—something beautiful, it is implied—in exchange for a constraint—something not beautiful, we understand—if it meant you could be free of grief—a form of pain only possible in the aftermath of something beautiful? Haunting each part of the equation is love.

Misapprehending the swirl of his body in the dark tangle of 6:00 A.M., I accidentally knee my son in the head as I sit down on the edge of his bed to wake him. Not gentle, the thud; gentle, the sleepy whimper. Always I can hear my mother's throat constricting when she answers my questions about the time I tumbled from a swing at the playground by the pond we used to go to in summertime and hit my head on something, a rock maybe, falling briefly unconscious.

I was very young, a toddler, elastic still, even to some extent of joint and of bone. I don't remember the fall or any pain. I remember the police car from the flashing inside as we drove to some nearby emergency room. They checked me out. Everything was fine. But every so often, probing for a deeper history, biased toward injury and convinced they'll find some more satisfying causality lurking there, the story pricks the ears of some new doctor or body worker and I have no choice but to stroll around with them in those narrative woods, no choice, every so often, but to ask my mother what they want to know of those trees.

The slight strangle doesn't enter her voice when we talk about family history. She had occasional migraines premenopause—visual aura plus pain, once or twice a year, triggered by sadness or stress and cured with coffee—"nothing like what you have," as she always says, but enough to make for a clear hereditary predisposition. Somehow more definitive yet easier to accept: the guilt of inheritance (fate) versus the guilt of accident (chance).

Almost immediately upon becoming pregnant, I realized I was already worried about dropping the baby. My partner would have to wait many months for the birth before such a thing would be possible for him, but already I faced off every minute of every day with a terrifying range of exigencies—some known, more unknown— hovering within and beyond my control.

Alongside the idea that we select for beauty, *Now Now Oh Now*'s heartbroken ornithologist argues for the role of chance. Not with as much passion, or with less embrace, that is, she argues for the beating heart of beauty but acknowledges the cold kiss of chance. The audience, each of us

seated around a magnificent table before a carefully laid place, is asked to roll the dice in front
of us. "A fire tears through this theater. Some of
us succumb; some of us survive," she says. "Look
at the dice before you. Evens, you're dead."

37

I no longer lie on couches trying to wrap my mind around the concept of infinity or apprehend through stillness passing parcels of unreproducible time, but in a more recent mental exercise I find myself wrestling with the riddle of causality. Preoccupied with the fact that there are, in fact, answers—theoretically at least—to many of the mysteries making up our lives, I fantasize a sort of forensic investigation/exposé companion program running alongside the day-to-day. Going macro, going micro, it would reveal, for instance, that this was the exact moment a virus passed from one person to another; these were the tiny fractions by which a valve loosened until it was free to blow; this sperm here out of the millions; this chromosome selecting; this DNA dividing, this moment in the cascade; this notch in the occipital ledge; this injury to the toddler's head.

Sometimes chance is cause, but is it ever what we mean by causality? Chance is cause stripped of meaning, an origin story or fated end without moral or lesson. ("People get what they get; it has nothing to do with what they deserve." [*House M.D.*]) But any cause as yet unknown glows luminous. Answerless, we search for answers, because questions call and press. Somewhere out there, we feel sure, is the information that means, but, beyond our reach, it can't matter yet. And when causality's riddle turns out to be procedural or a purely chance operation, can it ever?

Maybe it's a question of meaning versus meaningfulness. Chance may not teach us anything, but chance identified is a kind of answer and therefore a kind of balm, a version of no blame. I mean, in a way it's reassuring how clearly the migraines come and go of their own volition, according to their own logic. One way of translating the void, the reams of unilluminating data, the typically atypical patterns: there's nothing you did; there's nothing you can do.

"So what did you end up working on?" Cole asks over dinner a few weeks after I return, a present closer to the ever-sliding now. I wrote about pain, I say, that it feels strange to have done so. "You really don't let people know about that, do you?" he half-asks, half-assesses. "For instance, people at work." "I don't hide it," I say, "I can't if you know me well or see me every day, but in general I feel like it's no one's business." "People judge," he offers. "And people assume," I say. "Besides," I blurt out a little too loudly, "suffering is private."

5:00 A.M., blindered, desperate for the meds to kick in, I blink at a blinking screen. "Every day brings its own kind of education," Jane Goodall is saying, reflecting on the nature of experience. Later, I watch a video of animals being freed from cages of various kinds. Almost without fail, they step cautiously at first: the chimps hug and look up at the sky; the foxes and chickens both walk tentatively forward, pulling their feet high; the seals lurch, then slide; even the lion moves slowly; but the tiger shoots out like a flame.

38

"From out the inscrutable depths of nature myriads of dark effluences strike with subtle touch the attuned chords of our responsive being, and lo! the perceptible world, and we therein, stand revealed in the conscious medium of vivid sensations and perceptions," wrote the Scottish-born physician Dr. Edmund Duncan Montgomery in a paper titled "Are We Conscious Automata," delivered to the Texas Academy of Science in 1896.

"I see the trees as gallery walls, the wind as collaborator," says the artist Nancy Mims to the small crowd assembled on the lawn outside the museum, among the breeze-billowing photographs of flowers printed large-scale on soft canvas and hung from trees. "Each flower is its own fleeting moment of beauty at the cusp of decay," she continues. Some are cut into narrow strips and woven piece by piece back into a whole—now newly textured, like and unlike, collaged and quilted—on string-suspended looms affixed like spiderwebs between trunks.

This was the art I meant to see. I only stumbled upon Montgomery accidentally inside the museum I didn't intend to enter, in a tiny tower room put there by his wife, the sculptor Elisabet Ney, for him to read and write in while she carved snow-white marble below, to which I climbed only to humor the boy I'd dragged along. "We, the children of fulfilling Fate, with open heart and ready will, are soliciting for our all-evolving Mother some little insight into the true meaning of the life we bear."

Patient during his weeks of debilitation, cautious during the slow months of his recovery, now the cat navigates seemingly seamlessly according to the revised physics of his body in space. He leaps a little. He more often levers than leaps. Somehow, he finds a way to break his leaps down into manageable portions, sequences of smaller affairs. Just as then, car-struck, he found a way to make it home with two wrecked hind legs, dragging a belly blooming crimson. Just as now he finds a way, board by board, to scale the tall wooden fence.

Maybe red—plush of body deep inside or just beneath the surface, plush of blood—gets as much play? It's hard to say. Attention is a rigged divining rod. Anyway, blood half the time, we were taught—erroneously, it turns out, but cannot unsee—is blue.

Blue belongs to water and to sky equally, which is to say neither, after all. It belongs to us. That distant cleft between rises could be filled with sea, but isn't. What I thought was a wasp's mud nest docked on the front porch light is actually a swallow's. I only discovered it by lying on the living room floor. I only realized my mistake by lying there so long.

"The irony is that my catharsis was writing down that there is no catharsis," Maggie Nelson says in a recent interview. "The stories we tell ourselves don't heal us, but I also think that if I hadn't written it, I wouldn't have processed the experience."

And later: "I think of ideas as murmuring things you have to let talk to you in a quiet room."

Not writing about them didn't make them go away. Writing about them doesn't, either. Asked when she last heard the voice come to her, Joan answered, "I heard it yesterday and today." The truth is, sometimes I'm as if in a trance. The truth is entranced. (Horse, then, unhorses.)

> *she heard a voice*
>
> *she heard a voice on her right*
>
> *she often heard the voice*
>
> *she seldom hears it without the light*
>
> *the light comes from the same side*
>
> *around noon in summer*
>
> *in a wood she would*
>
> *in that place there is a great light*
>
> *the light was at her side*
>
> *she knew it was the voice*
>
> *she understood the voice well*
>
> *the voice told her to come*

the voice told her that she must

the voice told her that she, Joan, must

it was just as the voice had told her

(she was about to mount her horse when she answered)

Acknowledgments

I'm deeply indebted to the individuals and institutions whose encouragement and support was invaluable to me while writing this book:

Thank you to Martha Jessup, Douglas Humble, and the Lannan Foundation for the incomparable gift of a Writing Residency; to Rob Weiner and the Chinati Foundation for exquisite access to the sheds; to Oliver Franklin and the Elisabeth Ney Museum's Writer in Residence program for several fine weeks in a windy turret; and to the University of Texas at Austin's Faculty Research Award program for time off from teaching in which to write.

Thank you to Mary Szybist, first reader, visible and invisible companion throughout; to Elizabeth McCracken, final reader, whose advice made everything smarter and more possible; and to Eula Biss, Julie Carr, Jane Miller, Deborah Paredez, Srikanth Reddy, and Vincent Scarpa whose insight and enthusiasm were crucial along the way. Thanks, too, to the additional friends who offered helpful input on the manuscript in-process and/or essential companionship to the life in-progress: Heather Abel, Edward Carey, Rob Casper, Kris Delmhorst, Lauren Dias, Matthea Harvey, Noy Holland, Peter Kochansky, Cecily Parks, Barry Rothman, Petros Varthakouris, Michael Wiegers, and Matthew Zapruder.

Thank you to Margaret Babbot, Jill Heytens, Jeanne Hubbuch, Bill Ryan, Rivers Sterling, and Aline Zeringue for variously expert and unfailingly compassionate care.

Thank you to Erika Goldman, whose interest made this book a better version of itself, and to everyone at BLP for giving it such an excellent home.

And thank you most of all to my family, especially my parents, Linda and Michael Olstein, for a lifetime of love and support; to David for half a lifetime (and counting) of the same; and to Toby for being the source of so much love, hilarity, and inspiration.

Bibliography

Books

Daudet, Alphonse. *In the Land of Pain*. Translated by Julian Barnes. New York: Vintage Classics, 2016.

Elliot, Lise. *What's Going On In There: How the Brain and Mind Develop in the First Five Years of Life*. New York: Bantam Books, 1999.

Freeman, Katherine. *Ancilla to the Pre-Socratic Philosophers*. Cambridge: Harvard University Press, 1948.

Gawande, Atul. *Being Mortal: Medicine and What Matters in the End*. New York: Picador, 2017.

Goethe, Johann Wolfgang von. *Theory of Colors*. Translated by Charles Lock Eastlake. Mineola, NY: Dover Publications, 2006.

Harris, H. S. *The Reign of the Whirlwind*. Toronto: York Space Institutional Repository, 1999.

Hobbins, Daniel, ed. and trans. *The Trial of Joan of Arc*. Cambridge: Harvard University Press, 2005.

Inwood, Brad, and L. P. Gerson, eds. and trans. *The Epicurus Reader*. Indianapolis: Hackett, 1994.

Kandinsky, Wassily. *Concerning the Spiritual in Art*.
    Translated by M. T. H. Sadler. Mineola, NY:
    Dover Publications, 1977.

Lehrer, Jonah. *How We Decide*. Boston: Houghton
    Mifflin Harcourt, 2009.

Noë, Alva. *Strange Tools: Art and Human Nature*.
    New York: Hill and Wang, 2015.

Pliny the Elder. *Natural History: A Selection*.
    Translated by John F. Healy. London: Penguin
    Books, 1991.

Sacks, Oliver. *Migraine*. New York: Vintage Books,
    1992.

Scarry, Elaine. *The Body in Pain*. New York: Oxford
    University Press, 1985.

Woolf, Virginia. *On Being Ill*. Ashfield, MA: Paris
    Press, 2002.

Articles and Essays

Abel, Heather. "How to Stop a Tsunami in Three
    Easy Steps." *The Last Word on Nothing*, August
    17, 2015.

Biss, Eula. "The Pain Scale." *Seneca Review* 35, no. 1
    (January 5, 2005).

Carson, Anne. "Variations on the Right to Remain
    Silent." *A Public Space*, issue 7 (2008).

Hustvedt, Siri. "Knausgaard Writes Like a Woman:
    On Gendered Literature and the Feminization of
    Feelings." *Literary Hub*, December 10, 2015.

Jackson, V. "Lyric." In *The Princeton Encyclopedia
    of Poetry and Poetics*. 4th ed. Edited by Roland
    Greene and Stephen Cushman. Princeton:
    Princeton University Press, 2012.

Keh, Andrew. "Kobe Bryant the Bard Earns Mostly Positive Reviews." *New York Times*, December 2, 2015.

Lee, John M. "Some Remarks on Writing Mathematical Proofs." University of Washington Mathematics Department. Available at https://sites.math.washington.edu/~lee/Writing/writing-proofs.pdf.

McMahon, Kathy. "Exploring Emotional Reactions to Peak Oil." *Resilience*, August 27, 2006.

Montgomery, Edmund Duncan. "Are We Conscious Automata?" *Proceedings of the Texas Academy of Science*, 1897. MSS 0050, box 1, folder 20. Edmund Montgomery and Elizabet Ney Collection. DeGolyer Library, Southern Methodist University, Dallas, TX.

Noah, Timothy. "Our American Cousin Revisited." *Slate*, February 24, 2009.

Osnos, Evan. "In the Land of the Possible." *The New Yorker*, December 22 and 29, 2014.

Ott, Katharine. "Ten Tips for Writing Mathematical Proofs." University of Kentucky Department of Mathematics. Available at http://www.ms.uky.edu/~kott/proof_help.pdf.

Sedley, David. "Lucretius." *The Stanford Encyclopedia of Philosophy*. Edited by Edward N. Zalta. Available at https://plato.stanford.edu/entries/lucretius/.

Warren, James. "Anaxagoras on Perception, Pleasure, and Pain." In *Oxford Studies in Ancient Philosophy*. Vol. 33. Oxford: Oxford University Press, 2007.

Willis, Elizabeth. "Notes from and on a Landscape: Hell, Fire, and Brimstone." *Evening Will Come: A Monthly Journal of Poetics* 42 (June 2014).

Interviews

Dunn, Greg. "Dazzling Images of the Brain Created by Neuroscientist-Artist." By Tanya Lewis. *LiveScience*, December 10, 2014.

Goodall, Jane. "Jane's Interview." By Yann Arthus-Bertrand. *HUMAN the movie*, September 11, 2015.

Nelson, Maggie. "There is no catharsis . . . the Stories We Tell Ourselves Don't Heal Us." By Rachel Cooke. *The Guardian*, May 21, 2017.

Niffenegger, Audrey. "In 'Ghostly,' Phantoms Provide an Omniscient Point of View." By Ari Shapiro. *All Things Considered*, National Public Radio, October 30, 2015.

Dramatic Works

House M.D. Created by David Shore. Fox Broadcasting, 2004–2012.

Rude Mechs Theater Ensemble. *Now Now Oh Now*. Austin, TX: The Off Center, December 3, 2015.

Poems

Bishop, Elizabeth. "Little Exercise." In *Elizabeth Bishop, The Collected Poems 1927–1979*. New York: Farrar Straus and Giroux, 1983.

Dickinson, Emily. "After great pain," "One need not be a chamber," and "The brain has corridors." In *The Poems of Emily Dickinson: Reading Edition*. Edited by Ralph W. Franklin. Cambridge: Belnap Press, 1998.

Reddy, Srikanth. "Pain Quizzes XXVI." In *Underworld Lit*. Seattle: Wave Books, 2019.

Wright, C. D. "In a Word, a World." In *The Poet, The Lion, Talking Pictures, El Farolito, A Wedding in St. Roch, The Big Box Store, The Warp in the Mirror, Spring, Midnights, Fire & All*. Port Townsend, WA: Copper Canyon Press, 2016.

Other

"Beaufort Wind Scale: Developed in 1805 by Sir Francis Beaufort, U.K. Royal Navy." Storm Prediction Center of the National Weather Service. Available at https://www.spc.noaa.gov/faq/tornado/beaufort.html.

The Chinati Foundation. "Donald Judd, 100 works in mill aluminum 1982–1986." Available at https://www.chinati.org/collection/donaldjudd.

Janus Films. "The Passion of Joan of Arc: Introductory Text." The Criterion Collection.

Neighmond, Patti. "Why Women Suffer More Migraines Than Men." *Morning Edition*, National Public Radio, April 16, 2012.

Turrell, James. *The Color Inside*, 2013. University of Texas at Austin.

Wikipedia, The Free Encyclopedia. "Boolean algebra."

Credits and Permissions

Pages 77–78

"Night Moves" Words and Music by Bob Seger.

Copyright © 1976 Gear Publishing Co.

Copyright Renewed All Rights Reserved Used by Permission

Reprinted by Permission of Hal Leonard LLC

Page 93

"I'm On Fire" by Bruce Springsteen.

Copyright © 1958 Bruce Springsteen (Global Music Rights). Reprinted by permission. International copyright secured. All rights reserved.

Page 117

Excerpt from "Little Exercise" from *Poems* by Elizabeth Bishop. Copyright © 2011 by The Alice H. Methfessel Trust. Publisher's Note and compilation copyright © 2011 by Farrar, Straus and Giroux. Reprinted by permission of Farrar, Straus and Giroux.

"Lisa Olstein's luminous meditation on pain winds around a beautifully curated series of artifacts. Bits of poetry, ancient medicine, brain science, television episodes, excerpts from the trial of Joan of Arc, and works of art support the spiderweb on which her insights hang like condensed mist. A fascinating, totally seductive read!"

—EULA BISS, author of *Notes from No Man's Land* and *On Immunity*

"Olstein's remarkable *Pain Studies* is a book built of brain and nerve and blood and heart, about what it means to live with pain. Irreverent and astute, synthesizing the personal and the historical, popular culture and poetry and visual art, *Pain Studies* will change how you think about living with a body in our beautiful and doomed world."

—ELIZABETH McCRACKEN, author of *Thunderstruck* and *Bowlaway*

"These spectacular sentences chart a thrilling investigation into pain, language, and Olstein's own exile from what Woolf called 'the army of the upright.' On a search path through art, science, poetry, and prime-time television, Olstein aims her knife-bright compassion at the very thing we're all running from. *Pain Studies* is a masterpiece."

—LENI ZUMAS, author of *The Listeners* and *Red Clocks*

In this extended lyric essay, a poet mines her lifelong experience with migraine to deliver a marvelously idiosyncratic cultural history of pain—how we experience, express, treat, and mistreat it. Her sources range from the trial of Joan of Arc to the essays of Virginia Woolf and Elaine Scarry to Hugh Laurie's portrayal of Gregory House on *House M.D.* As she engages with science, philosophy, visual art, rock lyrics, and field notes from her own medical adventures (both mainstream and alternative), she finds a way to express the often-indescribable experience of living with pain. Eschewing simple epiphanies, Olstein instead gives us a new language to contemplate and empathize with a fundamental aspect of the human condition.

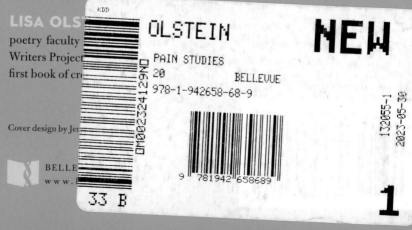

LISA OLS

poetry faculty

Writers Project

first book of cre

Cover design by Jer

BELLE
www.